Evidence-Based Pediatric Dentistry

Editor

DONALD L. CHI

DENTAL CLINICS OF NORTH AMERICA

www.dental.theclinics.com

July 2017 • Volume 61 • Number 3

ELSEVIER

1600 John F. Kennedy Boulevard • Suite 1800 • Philadelphia, Pennsylvania, 19103-2899

http://www.dental.theclinics.com

DENTAL CLINICS OF NORTH AMERICA Volume 61, Number 3
July 2017 ISSN 0011-8532, ISBN: 978-0-323-53128-3

Editor: John Vassallo; j.vassallo@elsevier.com
Developmental Editor: Kristen Helm

Dental Clinics of North America (ISSN 0011-8532) is published quarterly by Elsevier Inc., 360 Park Avenue South, New York, NY 10010-1710. Months of issue are January, April, July, and October. Business and Editorial Offices: 1600 John F. Kennedy Boulevard, Suite 1800, Philadelphia, PA 19103-2899. Periodicals postage paid at New York, NY and additional mailing offices. Subscription prices are $288.00 per year (domestic individuals), $569.00 per year (domestic institutions), $100.00 per year (domestic students/residents), $350.00 per year (Canadian individuals), $737.00 per year (Canadian institutions), $422.00 per year (international individuals), $737.00 per year (international institutions), and $200.00 per year (international and Canadian students/residents). International air speed delivery is included in all *Clinics* subscription prices. All prices are subject to change without notice. **POSTMASTER:** Send address changes to *Dental Clinics of North America*, Elsevier Health Sciences Division, Subscription Customer Service, 3251 Riverport Lane, Maryland Heights, MO 63043. **Customer Service (orders, claims, online, change of address): Elsevier Health Sciences Division, Subscription Customer Service, 3251 Riverport Lane, Maryland Heights, MO 63043. Tel: 1-800-654-2452 (U.S. and Canada). Fax: 314-447-8029. E-mail: journalscustomer service-usa@elsevier.com (for print support); journalsonlinesupport-usa@elsevier.com (for online support).**

Reprints. For copies of 100 or more, of articles in this publication, please contact the Commercial Reprints Department, Elsevier Inc., 360 Park Avenue South, New York, NY 10010-1710. Tel.: 212-633-3874; Fax: 212-633-3820; E-mail: reprints@elsevier.com.

The *Dental Clinics of North America* is covered in *MEDLINE/PubMed (Index Medicus), Current Contents/Clinical Medicine, ISI/BIOMED* and *Clinahl.*

Contributors

EDITOR

DONALD L. CHI, DDS, PhD
Associate Professor, Department of Oral Health Sciences, School of Dentistry, University of Washington, Seattle, Washington; Fellow, Center for Advanced Study in the Behavioral Sciences (CASBS), Stanford University, Palo Alto, California

AUTHORS

JUDITH ALBINO, PhD
President Emerita and Professor, Director, Center for Native Oral Health Research, Leadership for Innovative Team Science Program, Director, Colorado Clinical and Translational Sciences Institute, University of Colorado Anschutz Medical Campus, Aurora, Colorado

DAVID AVENETTI, DDS, MSD, MPH
Clinical Assistant Professor and Graduate Program Director, Department of Pediatric Dentistry, College of Dentistry, University of Illinois at Chicago, Chicago, Illinois

DONALD L. CHI, DDS, PhD
Associate Professor, Department of Oral Health Sciences, School of Dentistry, University of Washington, Seattle, Washington; Fellow, Center for Advanced Study in the Behavioral Sciences (CASBS), Stanford University, Palo Alto, California

STEPHANIE CRUZ, MA
Graduate Researcher, Department of Oral Health Sciences, School of Dentistry, University of Washington, Seattle, Washington

MARCIO A. DA FONSECA, DDS, MS
Associate Professor and Head, Department of Pediatric Dentistry, College of Dentistry, University of Illinois at Chicago, Chicago, Illinois

KIMON DIVARIS, DDS, PhD
Associate Professor, Department of Pediatric Dentistry, UNC School of Dentistry; Department of Epidemiology, Gillings School of Global Public Health, University of North Carolina at Chapel Hill, Chapel Hill, North Carolina

BURTON L. EDELSTEIN, DDS, MPH
Professor of Dental Medicine and Policy & Management, Columbia University Medical Center, Chair, Section of Population Oral Health, Columbia University College of Dental Medicine, New York, New York; Senior Fellow in Public Policy, Children's Dental Health Project, Washington, DC

IVETTE ESTRADA, MA, MPhil
Project Coordinator, Section of Population Oral Health, Columbia University College of Dental Medicine, New York, New York

TRACY L. FINLAYSON, PhD
Associate Professor, Division of Health Management and Policy, Graduate School of Public Health and Core Investigator, Institute for Behavioral and Community Health, San Diego State University, San Diego, California

PAUL GLASSMAN, DDS, MA, MBA
Professor of Dental Practice, Director, Community Oral Health, Director, Pacific Center for Special Care, University of the Pacific Arthur A. Dugoni School of Dentistry, San Francisco, California

ARIEL P. GREENBLATT, DMD, MPH
Project Director, Department of Epidemiology & Health Promotion, New York University College of Dentistry, New York, New York

AARTI GUPTA, BDS
Research Assistant, Institute for Behavioral and Community Health, San Diego, California

HIROKO IIDA, DDS, MPH
Director, New York State Oral Health Center of Excellence, Rochester, New York

CAROL KUNZEL, PhD
Department of Sociomedical Sciences, Columbia University Mailman School of Public Health, Associate Professor of Community Dentistry and Sociomedical Sciences at CUMC, Section of Population Oral Health, Columbia University College of Dental Medicine, New York, New York

ELIZABETH MERTZ, PhD, MA
Associate Professor, Preventive and Restorative Dental Sciences, Healthforce Center, University of California, San Francisco, San Francisco, California

SARA S. METCALF, PhD
Associate Professor, Department of Geography, The State University of New York at Buffalo, Buffalo, New York

JEAN MOORE, DrPH, MSN
Director, Center for Health Workforce Studies, School of Public Health, University at Albany, State University of New York, Rensselaer, New York

MARY E. NORTHRIDGE, PhD, MPH
Associate Professor, Department of Epidemiology & Health Promotion, New York University College of Dentistry, Professor of Clinical Sociomedical Sciences (in Dental Medicine), Department of Sociomedical Sciences, Columbia University Mailman School of Public Health, New York, New York

FRANCISCO J. RAMOS-GOMEZ, DDS, MS, MPH
Professor, Section of Pediatric Dentistry, University of California Los Angeles (UCLA) School of Dentistry, Los Angeles, California

ERIC W. SCHRIMSHAW, PhD
Associate Professor, Department of Sociomedical Sciences, Columbia University Mailman School of Public Health, New York, New York

JOANNE SPETZ, PhD
Professor, Philip R. Lee Institute for Health Policy Studies, Healthforce Center, University of California, San Francisco, San Francisco, California

TAMANNA TIWARI, MPH, MDS, BDS
Assistant Professor, Clinical Instructor, Department of Applied Dentistry, School of Dental Medicine, University of Colorado Anschutz Medical Campus, Aurora, Colorado

Contents

Preface: The Science and Art of Evidence-Based Pediatric Dentistry xi

Donald L. Chi

Oral Health Interventions During Pregnancy 467

Hiroko Iida

Oral health is a fundamental component of health and physical and mental well-being. Oral health is influenced by an individual's physiologic and psychosocial attributes and cumulative oral health experiences. The perinatal period is a critical time when health and oral health determinants set in and thus an important time for intervention. Recognition of the importance of oral health intervention during pregnancy and oral health infrastructures have substantially grown over the last several years. This article reviews the current state of knowledge and practice of oral health intervention during pregnancy with a focus on individual- and population-based strategies, and summarizes key agendas for advancing prenatal oral health.

Prenatal Maternal Factors, Intergenerational Transmission of Disease, and Child Oral Health Outcomes 483

Tracy L. Finlayson, Aarti Gupta, and Francisco J. Ramos-Gomez

This article reviews maternal prenatal risk factors for caries in children and intergenerational transmission of caries, emphasizing early interventions for pregnant women and mother-infant pairs. A growing body of evidence focuses on maternal interventions. Studies suggest that early prenatal clinical and educational interventions are effective at reducing mother-child mutans streptococci (MS) transmission and delaying colonization and caries in young children. Dental screenings and anticipatory guidance about maternal and infant oral health should be included in prenatal care and pediatric well visits. Dental care during pregnancy is safe and recommended and can reduce maternal MS levels. Infants should visit a dentist by age 1.

Social Determinants of Pediatric Oral Health 519

Marcio A. da Fonseca and David Avenetti

Social determinants of health are defined as conditions in which people are born and live and the role these conditions play on health outcomes. Research indicates that risk factors and their interactions are far more complex than originally thought. This article outlines social determinant constructs and their role in understanding oral health promotion. Due to the complex interactions, oral health must be promoted using a multilevel chronic disease model or common risk factor approach. An understanding of social determinants is particularly important for the pediatric population because optimum oral health and general health in adulthood are heavily influenced by childhood.

Intergenerational and Social Interventions to Improve Children's Oral Health 533

Mary E. Northridge, Eric W. Schrimshaw, Ivette Estrada, Ariel P. Greenblatt, Sara S. Metcalf, and Carol Kunzel

Dental caries and gingival and periodontal diseases are commonly occurring, preventable chronic conditions in children. These diseases are more common in disadvantaged communities and marginalized populations. Thus, public health approaches that stress prevention are key to improving oral health equity. There is currently limited evidence on which community-based, population-level interventions are most effective and equitable in promoting children's oral health. More rigorous measurement and reporting of study findings are needed to improve the quality of available evidence. Improved understanding of the multilevel influences of children's oral health may lead to the design of more effective and equitable social interventions.

Acculturation and Pediatric Minority Oral Health Interventions 549

Tamanna Tiwari and Judith Albino

Immigrant populations are growing at a fast pace in the United States. Cultural variations can have implications on oral health of children from immigrant households. Length of stay in the United States and language spoken at home, proxies for measuring acculturation, are some of the crucial factors determining the level of acculturation in families. Higher acculturation generally has a positive impact on oral health utilization. Improving cultural competency of dental teams and involving the stakeholders in intervention design and implementation are some strategies that may increase the trust of ethnic minority patients and reduce barriers to access to care.

Interventions Focusing on Children with Special Health Care Needs 565

Paul Glassman

The term children with special health care needs encompasses a wide variety of conditions. When considering interventions, a broad definition of children with special needs is suggested in this article along with a focus on developing specific treatment recommendations based on a thorough data-gathering process and developing customized recommendations for children based on their unique circumstances. An area for future research is increasing the understanding of the relationship between customized recommendations and the underlying special health care needs.

Pediatric Workforce Issues 577

Elizabeth Mertz, Joanne Spetz, and Jean Moore

Untreated dental disease remains one of the most prevalent health conditions for children, driven in part by disparities in access to care. This article examines evidence-based workforce strategies being used to facilitate better access to pediatric health services and to improve oral health status and outcomes for children. The workforce strategies described in this article include promising new models in the dental field, with new and existing providers as well as emerging workforce models outside of the dental field. Case studies for some of these workforce strategies are also presented. Future directions and health policy implications are considered.

Pediatric Dental-Focused Interprofessional Interventions: Rethinking Early
Childhood Oral Health Management   589

Burton L. Edelstein

> Evidence of effectiveness for prevention of early childhood caries sug-
> gests that parent engagement needs to occur perinatally and that uncon-
> ventional providers, helping professionals like social workers and dietitians
> and lay health workers like community health workers, are most effective.
> This finding, coupled with the emergence of population-based account-
> able care, value-based purchasing with global payments, understanding
> of common risk factors for multiple conditions, and social determinants
> of health behaviors, calls for a rethinking of early childhood oral health
> care. A population-based model that incorporates unconventional pro-
> viders is suggested together with research needed to achieve caries re-
> ductions in at-risk families.

Parent Refusal of Topical Fluoride for Their Children: Clinical Strategies and
Future Research Priorities to Improve Evidence-Based Pediatric Dental Practice   607

Donald L. Chi

> A growing number of parents are refusing topical fluoride for their children
> during preventive dental and medical visits. This nascent clinical and pub-
> lic health problem warrants attention from dental professionals and the sci-
> entific community. Clinical and community-based strategies are available
> to improve fluoride-related communications with parents and the public. In
> terms of future research priorities, there is a need to develop screening
> tools to identify parents who are likely to refuse topical fluoride and diag-
> nostic instruments to uncover the reasons for topical fluoride refusal. This
> knowledge will lead to evidence-based strategies that can be widely
> disseminated into clinical practice.

Precision Dentistry in Early Childhood: The Central Role of Genomics   619

Kimon Divaris

> Pediatric oral health is determined by the interaction of environmental
> factors and genetic influences. This is the case for early childhood caries,
> the most common disease of childhood. The complexity of exogenous-
> environmental factors interacting with innate biological predispositions re-
> sults in a continuum of normal variation, as well as oral health and disease
> outcomes. Optimal oral health and care or precision dentistry warrants
> comprehensive understanding of these influences and tools enabling inter-
> vention on modifiable factors. This article reviews the current knowledge of
> the genomic basis of pediatric oral health and highlights known and postu-
> lated mechanistic pathways of action relevant to early childhood caries.

Research Evidence Use in Early and Periodic Screening, Diagnostic, and
Treatment Dental Medicaid Class Action Lawsuits   627

Stephanie Cruz and Donald L. Chi

> Little is known about research evidence use in dental Medicaid class ac-
> tion lawsuits. This qualitative study develops a conceptual model to under-
> stand the role of dentists and how research evidence was used. Archival
> analyses were conducted and 15 key informants interviewed. Dentists

had key roles requiring scientific expertise or clinical experience serving vulnerable populations. Most evidence was newly generated, not based on existing sources. Dentists were involved in all phases of the lawsuits. Future research should identify conditions fostering research evidence use in dental Medicaid lawsuits and whether high-quality research evidence use improves child health outcomes.

Index   **645**

DENTAL CLINICS OF NORTH AMERICA

FORTHCOMING ISSUES

October 2017
Dental Biomaterials
Jack Ferracane, Luiz E. Bertassoni, and
Carmem S. Pfeifer, *Editors*

January 2018
Dental Public Health
Michelle Henshaw and Astha Singhal,
Editors

April 2018
Oral Cancer
Eric T. Stoopler and Thomas P. Sollecito,
Editors

RECENT ISSUES

April 2017
Clinical Microbiology for the General Dentist
Arvind Babu Rajendra Santosh and
Orrett E. Ogle, *Editors*

January 2017
Endodontics: Clinical and Scientific Updates
Mo K. Kang, *Editor*

October 2016
**Impact of Oral Health on Interprofessional
Collaborative Practice**
Linda M. Kaste and Leslie R. Halpern,
Editors

ISSUE OF RELATED INTEREST

Oral and Maxillofacial Surgery Clinics of North America
November 2016 (Vol. 28, No. 4)
Coagulopathy
Jeffrey D. Bennett and Elie M. Ferneini, *Editors*
Available at: www.oralmaxsurgery.theclinics.com

THE CLINICS ARE AVAILABLE ONLINE!
Access your subscription at:
www.theclinics.com

Preface

The Science and Art of Evidence-Based Pediatric Dentistry

 CrossMark

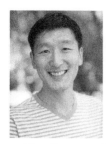

Donald L. Chi, DDS, PhD
Editor

Evidence-based pediatric dentistry involves a delicate balance between three factors: appropriate application of the best available science, craft knowledge accumulated through clinical experiences and patient values. The goal is to deliver care that optimize outcomes. Evidence-based dental practice is a value-free proposition: clinicians have the autonomy to make independent treatment and intervention decisions. This autonomy is bounded by an ethical obligation of nonmaleficence (do no harm) by keeping up-to-date on the relevant scientific literature that continues to expand, change, and evolve and is relevant in delivering the highest quality care.

The Internet has democratized science, making it easier for clinicians to communicate scientific literature, but barriers to science persist. There is a proliferation of basic, clinical, and translational studies in pediatric dentistry. Researchers from around the world are testing novel ideas and generating new knowledge, increasing the potential to transform disease prevention strategies, care delivery, and child health outcomes. Almost all studies are available online, some at no-cost through PubMed Central or Open Access. However, access to most publications costs money. A small number of clinicians affiliated with universities or hospitals can bypass these fees. Clinicians in practice are likely to search for free articles. Furthermore, assessing the quality of publications has become increasingly difficult, especially with the growing number of predatory journals and advertiser-sponsored articles that are free. These publications may not be peer-reviewed and may endorse commercial products of unknown quality or clinical approaches that are not evidence based. Thus, many clinicians have difficulties keeping current on the best available science, which is a significant barrier to evidence-based pediatric dental practice.

In this issue of the *Dental Clinics of North America*, our goal is to present trainees, clinicians, researchers, and policymakers with the most up-to-date science on

Dent Clin N Am 61 (2017) xi–xii
http://dx.doi.org/10.1016/j.cden.2017.04.001
0011-8532/17/© 2017 Published by Elsevier Inc.

dental.theclinics.com

important topics pertaining to pediatric dentistry. We highlight approaches for which there is empirical evidence and how the field can build on this knowledge.

In the first two articles, Iida and Finlayson and colleagues focus on prenatal and postnatal oral health interventions, with an emphasis on behavioral interventions, focusing on expectant and new mothers. Next, da Fonseca and Avenetti review the literature on the social determinants of pediatric oral health. Northridge and colleagues provide examples of intergenerational and social interventions aimed at improving pediatric health.

The next two articles focus on vulnerable populations. Tiwari and Albino review the literature on the effects of acculturation on the oral health of ethnic and racial minority children with an emphasis on evidence-based minority oral health interventions. Glassman focuses on children with special health care needs and reviews the methodologic challenges of classifying and identifying children who are in greatest need of interventions, focusing on disease prevention and management.

The pediatric dentistry workforce is at the frontline of implementing evidence-based practices and policies. Mertz and colleagues review the workforce literature with an emphasis on innovative evidence-based models of pediatric dental care delivery. Edelstein argues in favor of additional integration between pediatric dentistry and other related fields, including nutrition and social work, to address limitations of the existing workforce model.

The remaining articles highlight emerging issues in evidence-based pediatric dentistry. Chi describes the public health implications of topical fluoride refusal in pediatric dental practice, with emphases on clinical strategies and future research priorities. Divaris reviews the emerging literature on genomics and the potential for evidence-based precision dentistry approaches tailored to the profiles of children. Cruz and Chi examine two Medicaid dental class-action lawsuits to demonstrate how research evidence is used in the legal process and present a new conceptual model to help guide future evidence-based policymaking. We hope this issue will stimulate continued dialogue on how to improve the science and art of evidence-based pediatric dentistry.

Donald L. Chi, DDS, PhD
Department of Oral Health Sciences
School of Dentistry
University of Washington
Box 357475
B509 Health Sciences Building
Seattle, WA 98195-7475, USA

E-mail address:
dchi@uw.edu

Oral Health Interventions During Pregnancy

Hiroko Iida, DDS, MPH

KEYWORDS

- Oral health • Pregnancy • Perinatal health • Interventions

KEY POINTS

- Pregnancy is an ideal time to promote primary prevention of childhood oral diseases and oral health across the lifespan.
- Oral health and use of dental care during pregnancy are influenced by several factors surrounding pregnant women, health care, and finance systems.
- Promotion of oral health during pregnancy needs an evidence-based, multifaced, collaborative, and community-based approach to effectively address common risk factors and facilitate interoperable enabling and infrastructure-building maternal and child health services.

INTRODUCTION

Oral health intervention during pregnancy has attracted much attention in the context of perinatal maternal and child health over the last few decades. Pregnancy is an ideal time to promote primary prevention of oral diseases in children and convey the oral-systemic connection given the profound influence of maternal health and behaviors on children's oral health outcomes. Dental caries is a diet-dependent multifactorial bacterial disease, and studies show that maternal untreated caries and greater level of salivary cariogenic bacteria increase the odds of childhood caries.[1–5] Children's dietary and oral hygiene behaviors rely on parents or caregivers, and various psychosocial factors, such as caregivers' self-efficacy, oral health knowledge, and beliefs reportedly influence children's oral health and behaviors.[1,6–9] Primary teeth and some early erupting permanent teeth (permanent first molars and incisors) start to form during pregnancy; thus any complications and challenges during pregnancy and neonatal life may affect the optimal formation of enamel and caries risk in children.[1,10,11]

Adverse pregnancy outcomes, such as preterm birth, defined as a live birth before 37 weeks of gestation, and low birth weight (<2500 g or 5.5 pounds) occur 1 in 10 and

Disclosure Statement: The author does not have any commercial or financial conflict of interest.

New York State Oral Health Center of Excellence, 259 Monroe Avenue, Rochester, NY 14607, USA

E-mail address: hiida@rpcn.org

Dent Clin N Am 61 (2017) 467–481
http://dx.doi.org/10.1016/j.cden.2017.02.009
0011-8532/17/© 2017 Elsevier Inc. All rights reserved.

dental.theclinics.com

13 births in the United States, respectively, and are leading causes of early childhood mortality and morbidity.[12] Although the causes of adverse pregnancy outcomes are not well understood, bacterial infection and elevated levels of local and systemic markers of inflammation are linked to various pregnancy complications including preterm delivery.[13,14] Periodontitis is an infectious disease caused mainly by anaerobic gram-negative bacteria, which can induce a variety of inflammatory mediators, such as prostaglandins, interleukins, and tumor necrosis factor.[14] Because of hormonal and physioimmunologic changes many pregnant women experience progression of periodontal inflammation with increased vascular permeability, which can potentiate translocation of periodontal pathogens and/or their by-products to the fetal-placenta unit or trigger systemic inflammatory responses via the blood circulation.[13–15] Since the first report suggested a potential association between maternal periodontal infection and delivery of preterm and low-birth-weight infant in 1996,[16] many researchers examined this biologically plausible association. Despite the mixed evidence regarding the association between maternal periodontal health and birth outcomes,[17] periodontal disease shares common risk factors, such as maternal smoking, substance abuse, chronic health problems (ie, high blood pressure, diabetes, obesity), and low socioeconomic status with various pregnancy complications.[18,19] Oral health intervention during pregnancy is thus inarguably important from a life-course perspective to maternal and child oral health and overall health. This article reviews the current state of knowledge and practice of oral health intervention during pregnancy with a separate focus on individual- and population-based strategies and summarizes key agendas for advancing prenatal oral health.

INTERVENTION FOR INDIVIDUAL PREGNANT WOMAN
Caries Management and Control

Dental caries is a prevalent chronic disease among adults of reproductive age. About 82% of 20-to-34-year-old and 94% of 35-to-49-year-old US adults had caries experience during 2011 to 2012, and about 27% of them had untreated caries.[20] The rate of untreated caries was greater among adults of racial and ethnic minorities and was nearly twice as high among non-Hispanic black adults (42%) relative to non-Hispanic white adults (22%).[20] Changes in diet and oral hygiene practices and morning sickness or esophageal reflux during pregnancy can lead to tooth demineralization and thus an increase in maternal caries risk if appropriate interventions are not provided.[14] It has been documented that cariogenic microorganisms are often transmitted from intimate caregivers, usually mothers, to children.[21–24] Although significant colonization of cariogenic bacteria (ie, mutans streptococci [MS]) occurs after the eruption of teeth, it is reported that colonization of these microorganisms may occur from the time of birth.[22,23] It is essential therefore to promote maternal oral health during pregnancy through a dental home and risk-based oral health interventions.

Dental treatments, such as preventive, diagnostic, and restorative services, during pregnancy have not been associated with perinatal complications or medical adverse event.[14,25–27] The consequences of not treating an active disease process and infection during pregnancy outweigh the possible risk presented by most of the medications required for dental care.[25] Over the last decade, various national and state agencies have developed practice guidelines on oral health care for pregnant women (ie, the use of diagnostic radiation, restorative materials, management of patient behaviors and odontogenic infections, positioning pregnant patients during dental treatment, and dietary and oral hygiene instructions) to promote evidence-based oral health interventions during pregnancy (**Table 1**).[14,25,28] For some women, pregnancy

Table 1
National and state practice guidelines and policy statements on oral health care during pregnancy

Organizations	Guideline/Policy Documents	World Wide Web Link
Oral Health Care During Pregnancy Expert Workgroup (funded by the MCHB HRSA)	Oral Health Care During Pregnancy: A National Consensus Statement (2012)[28]	http://mchoralhealth.org/PDFs/ OralHealthPregnancyConsensus. pdf
Association of State and Territorial Dental Directors	Best Practice Approach: Perinatal Oral Health (2012)[1]	http://www.astdd.org/bestpractices/ BPAPernatalOralHhealth.pdf
American College of Obstetricians and Gynecologists	Oral Health Care During Pregnancy and Through the Lifespan: Committee Opinion (2013, reaffirmed 2015)	https://www.acog.org/-/media/ Committee-Opinions/Committee- on-Health-Care-for-Underserved- Women/co569.pdf? dmc=1&ts=20161004T1006239691
American Academy of Pediatric Dentistry	Guideline on Oral Health Care for the Pregnant Adolescent (2015/2016)	http://www.aapd.org/media/policies_ guidelines/g_pregnancy.pdf
	Guideline on Perinatal Oral Health Care (2015/2016)	http://www.aapd.org/media/policies_ guidelines/g_ perinataloralhealthcare.pdf
New York State Department of Health	Oral Health Care During Pregnancy and Early Childhood: Practice Guidelines (2006)[14]	http://www.health.ny.gov/ publications/0824.pdf
West Virginia University School of Dentistry	Oral Health Care During Pregnancy: At-a-Glance Reference Guide (2008)	http://mchoralhealth.org/PDFs/WV_ PregnancyRefGuide.pdf
University of Washington, Northwest Center to Reduce Oral Health Disparities	Guidelines for Oral Health Care in Pregnancy (2009)	http://depts.washington.edu/ nacrohd/sites/default/files/oral_ health_pregnancy_0.pdf
California Dental Association Foundation	Oral Health During Pregnancy and Early Childhood: Evidence-Based Guidelines for Health Professionals (2010)[25]	http://www.cdafoundation.org/ Portals/0/pdfs/poh_guidelines.pdf
South Carolina Oral Health Advisory Council and Coalition	Oral Health Care for Pregnant Women (2011)	http://www.scdhec.gov/library/CR- 009437.pdf
Maryland Department of Health and Mental Hygiene	Oral Health Care During Pregnancy: At-a-Glance Reference Guide (2012)	http://phpa.dhmh.maryland.gov/ oralhealth/docs1/pregnant_ women_reference_guide.pdf
Connecticut State Dental Association	Considerations for Dental Treatment of Pregnant Women: A Resource for Connecticut Dentists (2013)	http://www.csda.com/docs/default- source/dental-resources/ considerations-for-treating- pregnant-patients.pdf?sfvrsn=2

(continued on next page)

Organizations	Guideline/Policy Documents	World Wide Web Link
Michigan Department of Health and Human Services	During Pregnancy, the Mouth Matters: A Guide to Michigan Perinatal Oral Health (2015)	http://www.michigan.gov/documents/ mdhhs/Oral_Health_Guidelines_ 2015_508090_7.pdf
Massachusetts Department of Public Health	Massachusetts Oral Health Guidelines For Pregnancy and Early Childhood (2016)	http://www.mass.gov/eohhs/docs/ dph/com-health/data-translation/ oral-health-guidelines.pdf

Table 1
(continued)

Abbreviations: HRSA, Health Resources and Services Administration; MCHB, Maternal and Child Health Bureau of HRSA.

may be the only time they have dental insurance, thus dental providers may strategically sequence dental treatments based on patient's needs while putting elimination and control of etiologic factors and enhancing protective factors as the priorities.

There are several antimicrobial agents (ie, fluoride, chlorhexidine, iodine, xylitol, silver compounds) that have been studied to suppress cariogenic microorganisms and reduce caries experience.[29,30] Accumulated evidence, despite the high degree of heterogeneity and risk of bias, indicates that maternal habitual consumption of xylitol gums may reduce mother-child transmission of MS and delay the acquisition of MS in their children during early childhood.[29,31] The long-term effect of maternal xylitol gum exposure on their children's dental caries, however, is yet to be established.[19,31] In addition, the reported doses and frequencies of daily maternal consumption of xylitol that affect MS colonization in offspring vary significantly between studies (1–10 g/day, two to four times consumptions per day).[29,31] Nevertheless, the most critical factor to make this intervention work in the real world is the level of maternal adherence to the recommended regimen of xylitol consumption.

Community water fluoridation, a population-based caries intervention strategy that has been shown to be safe and cost-effective to reduce caries experience in the community, regardless of individual health behavior,[32,33] should be promoted by dental and prenatal health communities through coherent messages. Furthermore, dental and prenatal health care providers are in the best position to educate mothers-to-be about the evidence-based use of fluoride for the prevention of childhood caries reassuring its safety and allaying any potential misunderstandings.

The control and management of oral diseases highly depends on one's daily self-care and compliance to preventive and therapeutic measures.[34] Knowledge gain through conventional patient education, which focuses on disseminating information and giving normative advice, often does not translate into behavior changes.[34] In a collaborative counseling technique known as motivational interviewing (MI), clients assess their own behaviors, present arguments for change, and choose a behavior on which to focus through respectful questioning, reflection of ambivalence, and exploration of acceptable resolution.[34,35] MI has been used and evaluated to treat various lifestyle problems and chronic diseases including but not limited to tobacco smoking, substance abuse, obesity, and diabetes.[35] Systematic review and meta-analysis conducted by Borelli and colleagues[36] showed that parent-directed MI was associated with significant improvements in various pediatric health behaviors including oral health, such as tooth brushing and visiting the dentist relative to the comparison group. Although this finding on MI effect on pediatric oral health behaviors should be interpreted with caution because only small number of studies were available for synthetic data analyses, the data also suggested potential MI effect on reducing pediatric dental caries.[36]

Riedy and colleagues[37] tested the effect of two-phase (prenatal and postnatal) brief MI interventions on low-income mothers in rural Oregon and found no difference in the rates of maternal dental attendance during the perinatal period and their children's preventive dental visit by 18 months of age when compared with conventional health education. The authors found that most study participants were motivated to seek care and high-functioning at the baseline, and thus speculated that difference between the intervention groups in terms of psychosocial characteristics and the ability to keep and make dental appointments might have been small especially because patient navigator function was available to all participants.[37] Pregnancy is usually a time when women are motivated to adopt healthy behaviors for the unborn child. It is therefore an integral component of oral health intervention during pregnancy to successfully empower and guide women to adopt and sustain viable oral health behaviors for maternal and child oral health across the lifespan.

Management of Periodontal Health

Accumulated scientific evidence indicates that periodontal treatment during pregnancy, consisting of subgingival scaling and root planing, has no significant effect on preterm birth or birth weight, whereas the association of periodontitis and adverse birth outcomes and the effect of periodontal treatment may be greater among high-risk populations.[38–41] Despite the need of more evidence that improves clinical strategies to address periodontal disease in women during pregnancy, conventional periodontal therapy is reportedly associated with the improvement of maternal oral health during pregnancy.[26,42,43]

There have been substantial changes in the paradigm of clinical care departing from the traditional, procedure-driven care to a whole-person oriented, more integrated care that is accountable for the treatment outcomes over the last several years. Such an integrated approach is especially important for prevention and management of chronic diseases, such as periodontal disease and dental caries, which usually involve myriad environmental, behavioral, social, and biologic risk factors that determine the treatment outcomes. To better address periodontal disease in women of reproductive age, more evidence is needed to fill the knowledge gap regarding (1) appropriate case definition and treatment end point to monitor the periodontal health of women of reproductive age and evaluate the treatment outcomes, (2) etiologic pathogens that are potentially linked to adverse pregnancy outcomes, and (3) timing and strategies to better disrupt the etiologic pathway of periodontal disease in women of childbearing age.[13,15]

SYSTEM INTERVENTION FOR PRENATAL ORAL HEALTH

Despite heightened oral health needs and available intervention strategies to prevent and manage oral diseases, only 49%, 43%, and 48% of pregnant women reportedly visited a dentist, had their teeth cleaned, and received oral health advice on how to care for their teeth and gums during the most recent pregnancy, respectively, according to the 2011 Pregnancy Risk Assessment Monitoring System (PRAMS) data.[44] Among the same PRAMS survey participants, 56% reportedly had their teeth cleaned in the 12 months before pregnancy.[44] The use of dental care during pregnancy is influenced by several factors surrounding individual pregnant woman, health care, and finance systems. Because pregnant women may be uninformed or misinformed about the importance of oral health and/or lack personal resources to make a dental visit, oral health counseling, referral, and enabling services (ie, case management, care co-ordination/navigation, and outreach) should be available when women enter the pre-natal health care system. Such a multifaced, collaborative approach of prenatal oral health interventions would be a key to leverage limited resources in health care systems making more enabling services available for oral health; improve patient-centeredness, quality, safety, and outcomes of intervention; and make a sustainable impact to the oral health of maternal and child populations.

In 2006 New York State published the first of its kind perinatal oral health practice guidelines, which not only provided oral health recommendations for pregnant dental patients based on the scientific evidence and professional consensus but also drew a framework for interprofessional collaboration to improve access to oral health care during the perinatal period.[14] Other states and national agencies followed the foot-steps of New York State (see **Table 1**), and the landmark publication of the Oral Health Care During Pregnancy: A National Consensus Statement was made in 2012.[28] The release of this national consensus statement has promoted national, state, and local public health agencies to advocate and advance policy, resources, and workforce ca-pacity for perinatal oral health. As of 2014, a total of 16 states reportedly administered the oral health program for pregnant women,[45] and 22 states, District of Columbia (**Table 2**), and six territories/commonwealths (AS, FM, MP, MH, PR, VI) currently use the National Performance Measure 13A, "the percentage of women who had a dental visit during pregnancy," to assess the needs of maternal and child populations and evaluate the Title V Maternal and Child Health (MCH) Block Grant programs (see **Table 2**).[46,47]

The Maternal and Child Health Bureau of Health Resources and Services Adminis-tration in 2013 launched a multiyear national initiative, the Perinatal and Infant Oral Health Quality Improvement.[47] The goal of this initiative is to demonstrate the repli-cable, high-quality integration of oral health care into perinatal and infant primary care delivery systems with statewide reach and establish practice-based evidence to improve oral health of vulnerable maternal and child populations.[48] With the Peri-natal and Infant Oral Health Quality Improvement grant funding, a total of 15 states (see **Table 2**) are currently implementing various population-based intervention stra-tegies affecting health care and provider systems that impact access to and outcomes of perinatal oral health care especially among pregnant women and infants at risk for poor perinatal health and oral health outcomes.[48]

Workforce: Interprofessional Collaborative Training and Practice

Despite the clear benefit of promoting prenatal oral health, dental providers have been historically reluctant to provide dental care to pregnant women often postponing treat-ment until after giving birth. Meanwhile, prenatal health care providers generally have little prelicense education and training on oral health. The lack of professional consensus and competencies for prenatal oral health care and also a separation of professional education have resulted in poorly coordinated care to meet the oral health needs of vulnerable maternal and child populations.

It was not until recently that professional organizations and academia began to recognize the importance of interprofessional collaborative training and practices to promote safer and better, patient-centered, and community-oriented health care ser-vices. Workforce competency describes a set of professional knowledge, attitude, and skills required to work in a specialized area of profession, but the growing numbers of agencies concerning health professions education are now broadening

Table 2
Prenatal oral health infrastructure by state

State	Selection of NPM 13A[a,44-46] for MCH Title V Block Grant Program	PIOHQI[b,47]-Funded Program	State-Led Oral Health Program for Pregnant Women[45]	Medicaid/CHIP Income Eligibility Levels (FPL%) for Pregnant Women[45]	Medicaid Adult Benefits[c,59]	Medicaid Benefits for Pregnant Women[c,d,59]
AL	*					
AK				146	D,F,R,E,Ex,P,PM	
AZ		*	*	205		
AR				161	D,F,R,E,Ex,P,PM	D,F,R,E,Ex,P,PM
CA		*		214	D,F,R,E,Ex,PM	D,F,R,E,Ex,P,PM
CO		*		213	D,F,R,E,Ex,P,PM	D,F,R,E,Ex,P,PM
CT	*	*		200/265	D,F,R,E,Ex	D,F,R,E,Ex
DE	*			263		
DC	*		*	217	D,F,R,E,Ex,P,PM	D,F,R,E,Ex,P,PM
FL			*	211/324	D,Ex	D, Ex
GA	*		*	196	Ex	D,F,R,Ex,P,PM
HI	*			225	Ex	Ex
ID	*		*	196	D,F,R,E,Ex,P,PM	D,R,E,Ex,P,PM
IL	*		*	138	D,R,Ex	D,R,Ex,P
IN				213	D,R,E,Ex,P	D,R,E,ExP
IA	*		*	218	D,F,R,E,Ex,P,PM	D,F,R,E,Ex,P,PM
KS			*	380		
KY	*			171	D,R,Ex,P	D
				200		

(continued on next page)

Table 2
(continued)

State	Selection of NPM 13A[a,44-46] for MCH Title V Block Grant Program	PIOHQI[b,47]-Funded Program	State-Led Oral Health Program for Pregnant Women[45]	Medicaid/CHIP Income Eligibility Levels (FPL%) for Pregnant Women[45]	Medicaid Adult Benefits[c,59]	Medicaid Benefits for Pregnant Women[c,d,59]
LA				138	D	D
ME	*			214	R,E,Ex,P	
MD	*	*	*	264		D,F,R,E,Ex,P,PM
MA	*	*		205	D,R,Ex	
MI	*	*		200	D,R,Ex	D,R,Ex
MN	*	*		283	D,F,R,E,Ex,P	D
MS				199	Ex	Ex
MO				201	D,R,E,Ex,PM	D,R,E,Ex,P,PM
MT	*			162	D,F,R,E,Ex,PM	
NE			*	199	D,F,R,E,Ex,P,PM	D
NV				165	R,Ex,	D,R,Ex,P,PM
NH			*	201	Ex	Ex
NJ	*		*	199/205	D,F,R,E,Ex,P,PM	D,F,R,E,Ex,P,PM
NM		*		255	D,F,R,E,Ex,P	D,F,R,E,Ex,P
NY	*	*	*	223	D,F,R,E,Ex,P,PM	D,F,R,E,Ex,P,PM
NC				201	D,R,E,Ex,PM	D,R,E,Ex,PM
ND	*			152	D,F,R,E,Ex,P,PM	D,F,R,E,Ex,P,PM
OH				205	D,R,E,Ex	D,F,R,E,Ex

State		%			
OK	*	138		D,Ex	D,Ex
OR	*	190		D,F,R,E,Ex,P,PM	D,F,R,E,Ex,P,PM
PA	*	220		D,R,E,Ex,P,PM	D,R,E,Ex,P,PM
RI	*	195/258	*	D,R,E,Ex	D,R,E,Ex
SC	*	199	*	D,R,Ex	
SD	*	138			
TN		200			
TX	*	203	*		
UT	*	144	*	Ex	D,F,R,E,Ex,P
VT	*	213	*	D,F,R,E,Ex,P,PM	D,F,R,E,Ex,P,PM
VA		148/205	*	D,Ex	D,F,R,E,Ex,P,PM
WA		198		D,F,R,Ex,P,PM	D,F,R,Ex,P,PM
WV	*	163		Ex,PM	Ex,PM
WI	*	306	*	D,F,R,E,Ex,P,PM	D,F,R,E,Ex,P,PM
WY		159		D,F,R,Ex	D,F,R,Ex

Abbreviations: D, comprehensive examination (D0150) and/or periodic oral examination (D0120); E, endodontic treatment (D3220–3999); Ex, tooth extractions (D7140–7250); F, fluoride treatment (D1208) and/or fluoride varnish (D1206); FPL, federal poverty level; MCH, Maternal and Child Health; NPM, National Performance Measure; P, scaling and root planing (D4341–4342); PIOHQI, Perinatal and Infant Oral Health Quality Improvement; PM, periodontal maintenance (D4910); R, amalgam restorations (D2140–2161), and/or composite restorations (D2330–2394), and/or crowns (D2930–2954).

[a] The percentage of women who had a dental visit.

[b] The Perinatal and Infant Oral Health Quality Improvement Initiative, funded by the Maternal and Child Health Bureau, US Health Resources and Services Administration.

[c] 2014 MSDA Medicaid and CHIP oral health program survey data.

[d] Medicaid programs are required to provide "pregnancy related services and services or other conditions that might complicate pregnancy," during pregnancy and 60 days postpartum, for women up to 133% of FPL. Some states include dental benefits as part of these "pregnancy-related" services, regardless of whether they offer adult dental coverage.

the scope of competency reflecting the transformation and integration of health care systems.[49] For example, the Association of American Medical Colleges has developed several domains of oral health competencies for medical students, such as applying foundational knowledge of oral diseases and emergencies to perform basic assessment and screening of oral health, promotion of disease prevention and management, and collaborating with dental providers for optimal oral health and treatment outcomes.[50] The Commission of Dental Accreditation Standards state that dental students must be competent in providing oral health care in all stages of life and communicating and collaborating with other members of the health care team.[51,52]

To improve access to oral health services for vulnerable populations, Health Resources and Services Administration describes a core draft set of oral health clinical competencies (risk assessment, oral health evaluation, preventive interventions, communication and education, and interprofessional collaborative practice) for primary care providers who practice in safety net settings.[53] As of October 2016 there were nearly 51 million people living in more than 5000 dental health professional shortage areas across the country.[54] The shortage of dentists willing to treat pregnant women is compounded by geographic maldistribution of dentists and a shortage of dentists that participate in Medicaid program. Safety-net dental and primary care practitioners may be the critical players to address oral health needs of underserved mothers and their children during the perinatal period. The development of continuing education opportunities and the transformation of safety-net health care and finance system that support costs and competencies of prenatal oral health services are desperately needed. Furthermore, demonstration and evaluation of prelicense and postlicense provider trainings on prenatal oral health[52,55] would help refine the interprofessional collaborative approach to generate better and sustainable outcomes of prenatal oral health interventions and care coordination in the safety net systems.

Finance System

Various factors in dental finance systems, such as eligibility and coverage of dental benefits and availability and practice behavior of dental providers, affect oral health care during pregnancy. Pregnant women with incomes at or below 133% federal poverty level (FPL) have been a mandatory Medicaid eligibility group since 1989,[56] and all but four states have extended Medicaid coverage to pregnant women above the currently required level of 138% FPL under the Affordable Care Act in 2014 (see **Table 2**).[45] At present, more than half the states provide Medicaid eligibility for pregnant women with incomes up to at least 200% of the FPL (about $40,000 for a family of three in 2015),[45] and the Medicaid program finances almost half of all births.[56] Despite this extended health insurance coverage for pregnant women through public programs, adult dental benefits are optional Medicaid services, not a part of the essential health benefits requirement under the Affordable Care Act, thus always subject to being cut when states are under budget pressures. In addition, just as commercial dental plans typically do, many state Medicaid programs set a maximum on their per-person spending for adult dental benefits or impose caps on the number of certain services they cover (ie, one or two oral examinations and teeth cleanings a year).[57] Prior authorization is also commonly required for many dental services.[57] According to the data of national dental care expenditure in 2014, an overwhelming proportion of total dental expenditure ($113.5 billion) was financed by either private dental insurance (33%) or out-of-pocket spending (37%), and only 19% was financed by public programs.[58]

As of 2014, seven states provided no dental benefit and only 17 states provided comprehensive adult dental benefits, including diagnostic, preventive, some restorative and surgical services, and periodontal therapies under the adult Medicaid program (see **Table 2**).[59] There are two states that offered comprehensive dental benefits for pregnant women, whereas the adult beneficiaries had otherwise no or emergency-only dental benefits in 2014 (see **Table 2**).[59] In light of profound opportunity and importance of prenatal oral health intervention, policy makers should look at ways to expand eligibility and coverage of dental benefits for pregnant women, and to expedite the enrollment process and grant presumptive eligibility for pregnant women so that oral health needs of women would be properly and timely addressed during pregnancy. Furthermore, infrastructure for a value-based dental finance system, which incentivizes evidence-based clinical procedures that are accountable for the cost, quality, and outcomes of the MCH population, should be further explored over the coming decade.

SUMMARY

Oral health is a fundamental component of health and physical and mental well-being.[60] Over the life-course, oral health is influenced by an individual's physiologic and psychosocial attributes and cumulative oral health experiences. The perinatal period is a critical time when much of health and oral health determinants in children's lives set in, and thus is an important time for intervention. Recognition for the importance of oral health intervention during pregnancy and oral health infrastructures, such as data for strategic planning and evaluation, policies, and framework for system and service integration, to improve pregnant women's oral health have substantially grown over the last several years. Yet, there are gaps in resource and the knowledge base especially to improve oral health of vulnerable mothers and children. The following bullet points summarize the important action steps to advance prenatal oral health in the community. Each element is interrelated and requires an engagement of essential stakeholders in the public and private sectors, such as state and local governments, academic institutions, professional organizations, the MCH program, and dental providers and administrators:

- Improve access to quality prenatal oral health services:
  - Promote research to improve clinical strategies to address oral diseases and common risk factors in pregnant women
  - Promote interprofessional collaboration and make enabling services available to address oral health needs of pregnant women, especially those at risk for poor oral health and perinatal health outcomes
  - Evaluate existing prenatal oral health programs for quality improvement (ie, timeliness, safety, effectiveness, patient-centeredness, cost-efficiency, and equitability of oral health care and system- and process-barriers), and building practice-based evidence on prenatal oral health interventions
- Enhance national, state, and local infrastructure for oral health interventions during pregnancy:
  - Assess oral health needs, access, barriers, and disparities during pregnancy through PRAMS and/or other innovative data system (ie, safety-net administrative records) to monitor, plan, and evaluate prenatal oral health programs in the community
  - Enhance prelicense and postlicense collaborative training opportunities to develop and sustain prenatal oral health competencies among health care, dental, and support service providers

○ Build policy, finance, and technological infrastructure and provider networks that support prenatal oral health competencies, care coordination, and communication

○ Continue to transform health care and finance systems to be accountable for the outcomes of care, promote oral health and oral health–related quality of life across the lifespan, and capitalize interoperable resources to address oral health disparities

REFERENCES

1. Association of State and Territorial Dental Directors (ASTDD). Best practice approach. Sparks (NV): Perinatal Oral Health; 2012. Available at: http://www.astdd.org/bestpractices/BPAPernatalOralHhealth.pdf.

2. Smith RE, Badner VM, Morse DE, et al. Maternal risk indicators for childhood caries in an inner city population. Community Dent Oral Epidemiol 2002;30(3): 176–81.

3. Weintraub JA, Prakash P, Shain SG, et al. Mothers' caries increases odds of children's caries. J Dent Res 2010;89(9):954–8.

4. Dye BA, Vargas CM, Lee JJ, et al. Assessing the relationship between children's oral health status and that of their mothers. J Am Dent Assoc 2011;142(2): 173–83.

5. Chaffee BW, Gansky SA, Weintraub JA, et al. Maternal oral bacterial levels predict early childhood caries development. J Dent Res 2014;93(3):238–44.

6. Finlayson TL, Siefert K, Ismail AL, et al. Maternal self-efficacy and 1-5-year-old children's brushing habits. Community Dent Oral Epidemiol 2007;35(4):272–81.

7. Finlayson TL, Siefert K, Ismail AL, et al. Psychosocial factors and early childhood caries among low-income African-American children in Detroit. Community Dent Oral Epidemiol 2007;35(6):439–48.

8. Huebner CE, Riedy CA. Behavioral determinants of brushing young children's teeth: Implications for anticipatory guidance. Pediatr Dent 2010;32(1):48–55.

9. Wigen TI, Espelid I, Skaare AB, et al. Family characteristics and caries experience in preschool children. A longitudinal study from pregnancy to 5 years of age. Community Dent Oral Epidemiol 2011;39(4):311–7.

10. Lai PY, Seow WK, Tudehope DI, et al. Enamel hypoplasia and dental caries in very-low birthweight children: a case-controlled, longitudinal study. Pediatr Dent 1997;19(1):42–9.

11. Pascoe L, Seow WK. Enamel hypoplasia and dental caries in Australian aboriginal children: prevalence and correlation between the two disease. Pediatr Dent 1994;16(3):193–9.

12. US Department of Health and Human Services, Health Resources and Services Administration, Maternal and Child Health Bureau. Child health USA 2014. Preterm birth and low birth weight. Rockville (MD): U.S. Department of Health and Human Services; 2015. Available at: http://mchb.hrsa.gov/chusa14/health-status-behaviors/infants/pdf/preterm-birth-low-birth-weight.pdf.

13. Madianos PN, Bobetsis YA, Offenbacher S. Adverse pregnancy outcomes (APOs) and periodontal disease: pathogenic mechanisms. J Periodontol 2013; 84(4 Suppl):S170–80.

14. New York State Department of Health. Oral health care during pregnancy and early childhood: practice guidelines. Albany (NY): 2006. Available at: https://www.health.ny.gov/publications/0824.pdf. Accessed March 20, 2017.

15. Michalowicz BS, Gustafsson A, Thumbigere-Math V, et al. The effects of periodontal treatment on pregnancy outcomes. J Periodontol 2013;84(4 Suppl): S195–208.

16. Offenbacher S, Katz V, Fertik G, et al. Periodontal infection as a possible risk factor for preterm low birth weight. J Periodontol 1996;67:1103–13.

17. Ide M, Papapanou PN. Epidemiology of association between maternal periodontal disease and adverse pregnancy outcomes: systematic review. J Periodontol 2013;84(4 Suppl):S181–94.

18. Genco RJ, Borgnakke WS. Risk factors for periodontal disease. Periodontol 2000 2013;62(1):59–94.

19. National Institute of Child Health and Human Development. What are the factors that put a pregnancy at risk? Available at: https://www.nichd.nih.gov/health/topics/high-risk/conditioninfo/pages/factors.aspx. Accessed March 20, 2017.

20. Dye BA, Thornton-Evans G, Li X, et al. Dental caries and tooth loss in adults in the United States, 2011-12. NCHS Data Brief, No. 197. Hyattsville (MD): National Center for Health Statistics; 2015. Available at: https://www.cdc.gov/nchs/data/databriefs/db197.pdf.

21. Li Y, Caufield PW. The fidelity of initial acquisition of mutans streptococci by infants from their mothers;. J Dent Res 1995;74(2):681–5.

22. American Academy of Pediatric Dentistry. Guideline on infant oral health care. Pediatr Dent 2015-2016;37(6):146–50. Available at: http://www.aapd.org/media/policies_guidelines/g_infantoralhealthcare.pdf.

23. Berkowitz RJ. Mutans streptococci: acquisition and transmission. Pediatr Dent 2006;28(2):106–9.

24. da Silva Bastos Vde A, Freitas-Fernandes LB, Fidalgo TK, et al. Mother-to-child transmission of *Streptococcus mutans*: a systematic review and meta-analysis. J Dent 2015;43(2):181–91.

25. California Dental Foundation. Oral health during pregnancy and early childhood: evidence-based guidelines for health professionals. Sacramento (CA): 2010. Available at: http://www.cdafoundation.org/Portals/0/pdfs/poh_guidelines.pdf. Accessed March 20, 2017.

26. Offenbacher S, Beck JD, Jared HL, et al. Effects of periodontal therapy on rate of preterm delivery: a randomized controlled trial. Obstet Gynecol 2009;114(3): 551–9.

27. Michalowicz BS, DiAngelis AJ, Novak MJ, et al. Examining the safety of dental treatment in pregnant women. J Am Dent Assoc 2008;139(6):685–95.

28. Oral Health Care During Pregnancy Expert Workgroup. Oral health care during pregnancy: a national consensus statement. Washington, DC: National Maternal and Child Oral Health Resource Center; 2012. Available at: http://mchoralhealth.org/PDFs/OralHealthPregnancyConsensus.pdf.

29. Li Y, Tanner A. Effect of antimicrobial interventions on the oral microbiota associated with early childhood caries. Pediatr Dent 2015;37(3):226–44.

30. Featherstone JD, White JM, Hoover CI, et al. A randomized clinical trial of anti-caries therapies targeted according to risk assessment (caries management by risk assessment). Caries Res 2012;46(2):118–29.

31. Lin HK, Fang CE, Huang MS, et al. Effect of maternal use of chewing gums containing xylitol on transmission of mutans streptococci in children: a meta-analysis of randomized controlled trials. Int J Paediatr Dent 2016;26(1):35–44.

32. Community Preventive Services Task Force. Preventing dental caries: community water fluoridation. Available at: http://www.thecommunityguide.org/oral/fluoridation.html. Accessed March 20, 2017.

33. Murthy VH. Surgeon General's perspectives. Public Health Rep 2015;130(4): 296–8.

34. Gao X, Lo EC, Kot SC, et al. Motivational interviewing in improving oral health: a systematic review of randomized controlled trials. J Periodontol 2014;85(3): 426–37.

35. Rubak S, Sandbaek A, Lauritzen T, et al. Motivational interviewing: a systematic review and meta-analysis. Br J Gen Pract 2005;55(513):305–12.

36. Borrelli B, Tooley EM, Scott-Sheldon LA. Motivational interviewing for parent-child health interventions: a systematic review and meta-analysis. Pediatr Dent 2015; 37(3):254–65.

37. Riedy CA, Weinstein P, Mancl L, et al. Dental attendance among low-income women and their children following a brief motivational counseling intervention: a community randomized trial. Soc Sci Med 2015;144:9–18.

38. Schwendicke F, Karimbux N, Allareddy V, et al. Periodontal treatment for preventing adverse pregnancy outcomes: a meta- and trial sequential analysis. PLoS One 2015;19(6):e0129060.

39. Xiong X, Buekens P, Fraser WD, et al. Periodontal disease and adverse pregnancy outcomes: a systematic review. BJOG 2006;113(2):135–43.

40. Kim AJ, Lo AJ, Pullin DA, et al. Scaling and root planing treatment for periodontitis to reduce preterm birth and low birth weight: a systematic review and meta-analysis of randomized controlled trials. J Periodontol 2012;83(12):1508–19.

41. Polyzos NP, Polyzos IP, Zavos A, et al. Obstetric outcomes after treatment of periodontal disease during pregnancy: systematic review and meta-analysis. BMJ 2010;341:c7017.

42. Michalowicz BS, Hodges JS, DiAngelis AJ, et al. Treatment of periodontal disease and the risk of preterm birth. N Engl J Med 2006;355(18):1885–94.

43. Newnham JP, Newnham IA, Ball CM, et al. Treatment of periodontal disease during pregnancy: a randomized controlled trial. Obstet Gynecol 2009;114(6): 1239–48.

44. Centers for Disease Control and Prevention. PRAMStat System. Available at: http://www.cdc.gov/prams/pramstat/index.html. Accessed March 20, 2017.

45. Association of State and Territorial Dental Directors. FY 2014-15 State Dental Director Survey for the Synopses of State Dental Public Health Programs. 2016. Available at: http://www.astdd.org/. Accessed March 20, 2017.

46. Association of State and Territorial Dental Directors. MCH Title V National Performance Measure for Oral Health: Summary. Available at: http://www.astdd.org/docs/mch-npm-combined-summary-and-detailed-overview-03-20-2015.pdf. Accessed March 20, 2017.

47. National Maternal and Child Oral Health Resource Center. Promoting Oral Health During Pregnancy: Update on Activities—February 2016. Washington, DC. Available at: http://mchoralhealth.org/PDFs/OralHealthPregnancyUpdate_2_2016.pdf. Accessed March 20, 2017.

48. National Maternal and Child Oral Health Resource Center. Perinatal and Infant Oral Health Quality Improvement Initiative. Available at: http://mchoralhealth.org/projects/piohqi.php. Accessed March 20, 2017.

49. Interprofessional Education Collaborative Expert Panel. Core competencies for interprofessional collaborative practice: report of an expert panel. Washington, DC: Interprofessional Education Collaborative; 2011.

50. Association of American Medical Colleges. Oral health in medicine competencies for the undergraduate medical education curriculum. 2011. Available at: https://

www.mededportal.org/download/258096/data/ohicompetencies.pdf. Accessed March 20, 2017.

51. Commission on Dental Accreditation. Accreditation standards for dental education programs. 2013. Available at: http://www.ada.org/~/media/CODA/Files/predoc.ashx. Accessed March 20, 2017.

52. Jackson JT, Quinonez RB, Kerns AK, et al. Implementing a prenatal oral health program through interprofessional collaboration. J Dent Educ 2015;79(3):241–8.

53. US Department of Health and Human Services Health resources and Services Administration. Integration of Oral Health and Primary Care Practice. 2014. Available at: http://www.hrsa.gov/publichealth/clinical/oralhealth/primarycare/integrationoforalhealth.pdf. Accessed March 20, 2017.

54. Bureau of Health Workforce, Health Resources and Services Administration, US Department of Health and Human Services. Designated Health Professional Shortage Areas Statistics. 2016. Available at: C:/Users/hiida/Downloads/BCD_HPSA_SCR50_Smry.pdf. Accessed March 20, 2017.

55. Smiles for life: A national oral health curriculum. Course 5: Oral health for women: pregnancy and across the life span. Available at: http://www.smilesforlifeoralhealth.org/buildcontent.aspx?pagekey=101562&lastpagekey=101554&userkey=12604994&sessionkey=3066172&tut=555&customerkey=84&custsitegroupkey=0. Accessed March 20, 2017.

56. Paradise J, Lyons B, Rowland D. Medicaid at 50. Menlo Park (CA): The Henry J. Kaiser Family Foundation; 2015. Available at: http://files.kff.org/attachment/report-medicaid-at-50.

57. The Medicaid and CHIP Payment and Access Commission (MACPAC). Report to Congress on Medicaid and CHIP. Washington, DC: 2015. Available at: https://www.macpac.gov/wp-content/uploads/2015/06/June-2015-Report-to-Congress-on-Medicaid-and-CHIP.pdf. Accessed March 20, 2017.

58. Wall T, Vujicic M. US dental spending continues to be flat. Chicago: ADA Research Brief; 2015. Available at: http://www.ada.org/~/media/ADA/Science%20and%20Research/HPI/Files/HPIBrief_1215_2.ashx.

59. Medicaid Medicare CHIP Services Dental Association. National Profile of State Medicaid & CHIP Oral Health Programs. Available at: http://www.msdanationalprofile.com/. Accessed March 20, 2017.

60. US Department of Health and Human Services. Oral health in America: a report of the Surgeon General. Rockville (MD): US Department of Health and Human Services, National Institute of Dental and Craniofacial Research, National Institute of Health; 2000.

Prenatal Maternal Factors, Intergenerational Transmission of Disease, and Child Oral Health Outcomes

Tracy L. Finlayson, PhD[a],*, Aarti Gupta, BDS[b],
Francisco J. Ramos-Gomez, DDS, MS, MPH[c]

KEYWORDS

- Pregnancy • Prenatal/perinatal interventions • Early childhood caries/dental caries
- Bacteria transmission

KEY POINTS

- Interventions to reduce vertical bacterial transmission from mother to child to promote maternal and infant oral health should begin early, during pregnancy, or soon after delivery.
- Available evidence suggests that clinical and educational interventions beginning during pregnancy are effective at reducing mother-child mutans streptococci (MS) transmission and caries in young children.
- Evidence from maternal interventions after childbirth up to 24 months is more mixed, and more longitudinal oral health research is needed with pregnant mothers and mother-infant pairs postdelivery.
- Dental care is safe and recommended for pregnant women, and infants should have a first dental visit by age 1.
- Anticipatory guidance (AG) should be part of standard prenatal health care to promote maternal and infant oral health.

Disclosure Statement: The authors have nothing to disclose.
[a] Division of Health Management and Policy, Graduate School of Public Health, Institute for Behavioral and Community Health, San Diego State University, 9245 Sky Part Court, Suite 221, San Diego, CA 92123, USA; [b] Institute for Behavioral and Community Health, 9245 Sky Park Court, Suite 221, San Diego, CA 92123, USA; [c] Section of Pediatric Dentistry, University of California Los Angeles (UCLA) School of Dentistry, 10833 Le Conte Avenue, Box 951668, CHS Room 23-020B, Los Angeles, CA 90095-1668, USA
* Corresponding author.
E-mail address: tfinlays@mail.sdsu.edu

INTRODUCTION

Pregnancy is marked by multiple physiologic and other changes for mothers that affect their oral health.[1,2] Hormonal changes during pregnancy contribute to increased gingival inflammation, swelling, irritation, and pregnancy gingivitis.[3,4] Oral health problems, including dental caries, xerostomia, and greater tooth mobility, are also common during pregnancy.[5] The oral cavity can further be adversely affected from repeated vomiting during pregnancy, leading to possible perimylolysis. Maternal oral health during pregnancy and after childbirth also has implications for her infant's oral health.

This article reviews evidence of maternal prenatal risk factors for caries in children and intergenerational transmission of caries, emphasizing early interventions for women starting during pregnancy and within the first 24 months after the child is born. Promising strategies and future directions for improving clinical care for pregnant mothers and for mothers and infants are discussed.

EARLY CHILDHOOD CARIES

Dental caries in children up to 71 months old is considered early childhood caries (ECC).[6] ECC affects 23% of preschool-aged US children and is highly concentrated among children from low socioeconomic status (SES) backgrounds, racial/ethnic minorities, and immigrants.[7,8]

Multiple individual, family, and community-level factors are recognized as influencing ECC risk,[9] including maternal factors.[10–12] Mothers play a key role in shaping infant ECC risk.[13] Maternal oral health affects a child's ECC risk because cariogenic bacteria primarily pass from mother to child. The presence of certain oral microbes is needed for disease onset and progression. MS consists of several species, including *Streptococcus mutans* and *S sobrinus,* which are the primary oral bacteria responsible for ECC and found frequently in carious lesions.[14] MS colonization can happen shortly after birth[15]; thus, there is good reason to intervene early with pregnant mothers and infants.

PRENATAL FACTORS AFFECTING MATERNAL ORAL HEALTH AND INFANT EARLY CHILDHOOD CARIES RISK

Maternal oral health depends on biological, behavioral (personal oral hygiene, dental utilization, and health behaviors like smoking), and SES factors (cultural, psychosocial, and demographics).

Biological

Significant hormonal and immunologic changes make pregnant women more susceptible to oral health problems. In the United States, vital statistics report 15 years to 44 years as the reproductive/childbearing age range.[16,17] New mothers' mean age has shifted upward since 2000 to 26 years in 2014.[18] Developmental biological changes occur in this age range, independent of pregnancy changes. Younger pregnant adolescents may have good oral health but may still be physically developing themselves[19] and, as minors, may require parental consent before they can receive care, including dental treatment.[20] Furthermore, saliva composition and MS levels can change during pregnancy and postpartum, when mothers lactate.[1] Maternal prenatal oral bacteria levels have been shown to predict ECC.[21]

Behavioral

Most pregnant women (83%) report brushing twice daily and 24% report flossing daily.[22] Dental utilization during pregnancy varied by state between 1998 and 2006, from 25% to many reporting greater than 75%.[23–26] Prenatal smoking, higher prepregnancy weight, and no first-trimester prenatal care have been associated with enamel defects[27,28] and caries[29] in children.

Socioeconomic Status

SES disparities across clinical oral health indices exist among pregnant women,[30] and extensive problems have been documented among lower SES women while pregnant and postpartum.[31] In analysis of 1999 to 2004 National Health and Nutrition Examination Survey (NHANES) data, SES stratification showed that lower SES pregnant women had more untreated dental caries than nonpregnant women.[32] Mothers' lower SES and low educational attainment are associated with caries risk in young children.[12,33] Maternal psychosocial risk factors have also been associated with ECC and warrant further study.[34,35]

BACTERIA TRANSMISSION

Mother-to-child MS transmission is determined by a combination of maternal behaviors, MS virulence, and child host factors.[36]

Maternal Behaviors

Transmission of cariogenic bacteria occurs from primary caregivers, mostly from mothers, to young children,[37,38] through saliva.[39,40] Mothers with high MS (>10^5 colony-forming units [CFUs]/mL) are more likely to transfer bacteria to infants.[41] Infant MS colonization likelihood increases with close and frequent contact with the mother, through bottle or breastfeeding, pretasting food, and utensil sharing. Additionally, poor maternal oral hygiene, frequent snacking, and not cleaning a child's mouth after feeding further foster transmission.[42]

Mutans Streptococci Virulence

Oral microbiota is diverse. MS organisms vary in their ability to adhere to host surfaces. S mutans synthesize polysaccharides to produce acid, facilitating the ECC process.[15]

Child

Infants are susceptible to ECC before tooth eruption.[12] S mutans colonization can occur in predentate 3-month-old infants.[43,44] A window of infectivity period within the first 2 years of life overlapping with primary teeth eruption is when young children are most likely to acquire MS.[45] Earlier MS colonization significantly increases future caries risk.[39,46–48] Children with ECC are more likely to have caries later in life,[47,49,50] although longitudinal studies suggest it is possible for them to remain negative for MS with delayed colonization.[51]

METHOD

Prenatal and postdelivery maternal interventions (1998–2016) that focused on reduction of intergenerational MS transmission, child MS, and infant caries were reviewed (**Fig. 1**). Prenatal interventions were summarized separately from maternal interventions initiated at childbirth up to 24 months during an infant's window of infectivity to assess effectiveness of early interventions with mothers. Clinical outcomes of interest were maternal and/or infant MS reduction and infant ECC; 7 prenatal and 9

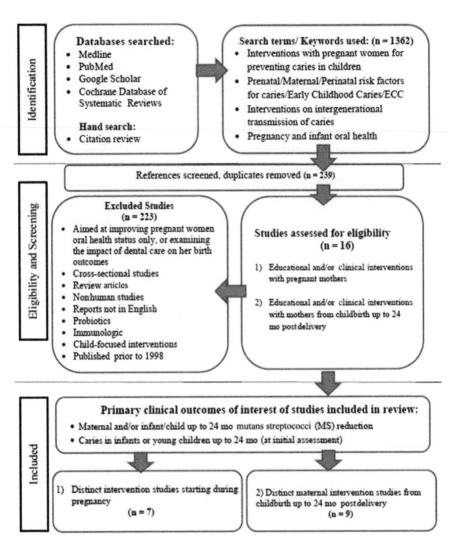

Fig. 1. Overview of the literature search and review method.

postdelivery maternal interventions met inclusion criteria. Cochrane systematic reviews of randomized controlled trials (RCTs) are currently under way on maternal xylitol use[52] and interventions with pregnant women and new mothers to prevent caries in their children.[53] For additional discussion of oral health interventions at the individual and population levels during pregnancy, see Hiroko Iida's article, "Oral Health Interventions During Pregnancy," in this issue.

Maternal interventions typically include education, AG, motivational interviewing (MI), dental care, and use of fluorides or antimicrobial agents to reduce MS levels. Alcohol-free rinses to reduce plaque and gingivitis are recommended during pregnancy, such as chlorhexidine (CHX) rinses.[54] Xylitol, a nonsugar sweetener used in foods, is also safe for pregnant women. Research indicates evidence of a dose-response effect,[55] with a total of 6 g/d dose consumed (specifically, 2g of xylitol, 3/d) recommended.

MATERNAL INTERVENTIONS
Prenatal

Table 1 summarizes 7 distinct prenatal intervention studies and their follow-up assessments.[56–67] One study focused on the impact of mothers chewing xylitol gum on child MS[60]; 4 studies focused on maternal education, treatment, and different antimicrobials on child caries[61–64] and MS.[65] Two education-only studies assessed child caries outcomes, after either MI[56] or repeated AG (printouts plus phone consultation).[66]

All antimicrobial prenatal studies were with high-MS mothers. Only 1 study tested xylitol gum chewing at recommended levels from pregnancy through 1 year. The intervention effectively reduced child MS levels at 24 months.[60] Furthermore, 23% of xylitol group children had reduced MS by 15 months postintervention.[58]

The 4 studies providing dental care and other antimicrobials to intervention groups found reduced child MS,[62–64] reduced maternal MS, and delayed children's MS colonization[65] and reductions in child caries.[59,61,67] Additional longitudinal studies with other high-risk and low-risk pregnant women are needed to confirm these findings on MS reduction and test linkages to children's caries outcomes.

Repeated AG during pregnancy resulted in reduced ECC incidence of test group children at age 2 compared with the control group (1.7% vs 9.6%).[66] Follow-up results also found reduced caries severity among test group children age 6 to 7 years[57] and provide evidence supporting the importance and impact of prenatal AG on reducing ECC. AG should be part of prenatal oral health programs. MI is more time intensive than AG, and no MI treatment effect was reported on caries rates overall.

In sum, there are too few and varied prenatal maternal interventions to draw firm conclusions about the evidence collectively. Reductions in maternal MS and child MS and child caries, however, were observed in 6 of the 7 studies. These are promising prenatal strategies for oral health promotion and infant caries prevention.

Postdelivery

Table 2 summarizes 9 distinct intervention studies and follow-ups. Four studies focused primarily on xylitol,[48,68–74] 2 studies tested CHX varnish,[75,76] 2 studies included preventive or restorative dental care plus CHX rinse,[77,78] and 1 study used an MI counseling approach.[79–81] Two studies did not assess the oral health status of the mother.[70,71,79,80] Outcomes for the interventions varied, including MS levels, plaque levels, and/or caries in the mother and/or child.

One xylitol lozenge study included anxious and nonanxious mothers and found that children in the xylitol intervention group had lower levels of caries.[73] The other 3 xylitol studies targeted mothers with high MS and had them chew gum.[48,68–74] One other xylitol intervention yielded significant changes in some outcomes of interest; although there was no reduction in maternal MS, few children in the maternal xylitol group had detectable levels of MS.[48] Longer-term effects were also reported in the 3-year and 5-year follow-ups.[68,69,82]

The 2 RCTs using CHX varnish over a 2-year period demonstrated significant impact on reducing maternal MS.[75,76] Only 1 study also assessed caries but found no differences in caries increment in mothers or children.[76] These findings suggest CHX varnish at regular intervals can reduce mothers' MS levels. Future maternal CHX varnish investigations should also include caries assessments and be conducted with larger samples.

The studies with dental care and CHX rinse also reported on MS levels and caries postintervention. One RCT reported short-term effects on maternal MS only after

Table 1
Summary of intervention studies by type with pregnant women to reduce mutans streptococci transmission and prevent caries in children (1998–2016)

Author, Year, Country	Study Length, Design, and Objective	Sample Characteristics	Intervention	Clinical Outcomes		Results
				Mother	Child	
Xylitol gum interventions						
Nakai et al,[60] 2010, Japan Shinga-Ishihara et al,[58] 2012	28-mo RCT to confirm the effectiveness of maternal early exposure to xylitol chewing gum on mother-child transmission of MS	Recruited women 3–5 mo pregnant with high MS. Randomized into 2 groups (n = 107), xylitol gum (xylitol; n = 56), and no gum (control; n = 51)	Both groups received the same preventive measures in the 6th mo of pregnancy: oral hygiene instruction and professional tooth cleaning. The xylitol group chewed 1 gum pellet (1.32 g) for ≥5 min at least 4 times/d starting at the 6th mo of pregnancy and terminated 13 mo later. No child in either group experienced any intervention. Children followed until age 24 mo	None	MS levels in children were assessed when the child was age 6 mo, 9 mo, 12 mo, 18 mo, and 24 mo.	77 Mother-child pairs at end of study. Mothers' mean xylitol frequency = 2.9×/d; mean dose = 3.83 g/d. Control group 8.8 mo earlier MS colonization than xylitol group Xylitol group less likely to be MS positive at 9 mo than control group

Preventive dental care, education, and antimicrobial agents: sodium fluoride and chlorhexidine component

Günay et al,[62] 1998, Germany; Meyer et al,[63] 2010; Meyer et al,[64] 2014	4-y prospective clinical long-term study to determine the effects of a prevention program on the oral health of children	Phase 1: intervention on 86 women during 3–4 mo of pregnancy. Phase 2: 54 mother-child pairs assessed, 0–3 y of age. Controls = 65	The entire study was subdivided into 5 phases. The first phase started during pregnancy and was continued in the 2nd phase for mothers/babies (0–3 y) and extended into a 3rd phase for mothers/preschool children (4–6 y). All 3 phases composed of an individual examination, preventive and need-related restorative treatment, topical FV application, CHX rinsing along with education and diet counseling both for mother and infant every 6 mo until 3 y and every 12 mo until 6 y of age.	MS levels, DF-S/DMFT, CPITN, API	dmfs, API, salivary level of MS	There were significant reductions in MS score and MS levels in saliva for both mothers and children. Additionally all mothers revealed a significant improvement in oral health. Prenatal and postnatal preventive programs may significantly improve the oral health of mothers and their children.

(continued on next page)

Table 1
(continued)

Author, Year, Country	Study Length, Design, and Objective	Sample Characteristics	Intervention	Clinical Outcomes		Results
				Mother	Child	
Gomez & Weber,[59] 2001, Chile Gomez et al,[67] 2001	Prospective clinical long-term study to evaluate if a preventive dental program, which started in pregnant women and continued postnatally, would be effective for a long-term reduction of dental caries	241 Mothers during 4 mo of pregnancy for intervention and 180 children of these selected randomly between 1 and 3.5 y of age for evaluation Control group — 180 children same age range randomly selected	Preventive dental program conducted simultaneously with obstetric visit; 3 parts: 1. Initial examination for pregnant mother and later their children 2. An educational part aimed at mothers about oral hygiene and dietary habits 3. A preventive and restorative treatment part for mother and antimicrobial mouth rinse at home	None	dft	Significant differences in caries status between groups. After 4 y, 97% intervention children caries-free compared with 77% in control group.

Source	Purpose	Sample	Methods	Outcome Measures		Results
Brambilla et al,[65] 1998, Italy	Prospective observational study to evaluate whether the reduction of salivary MS levels in a sample of highly infected women via a minimal preventive regimen during pregnancy could influence the mother-to-child transmission of this organism	65 High-MS mothers recruited at end of 6 mo of pregnancy until delivery Randomized into 2 groups: experimental and control	Both groups: dietary counseling, 1 session of professional prophylaxis along with oral hygiene instructions and use of systemic fluoride (1 mg of fluoride/d) For experimental group, subjects rinsed daily with 0.05% NaF and 0.12% CHX with two 10-d rinse-free intervals Both groups began treatment at the end of the 6th mo of pregnancy and continued until about the time of delivery.	Levels of MS (unstimulated saliva in sterile plastic pipette)	MS levels (unstimulated saliva in sterile plastic pipette)	Over the 30-mo study period, the NaF and CHX treatment regimens significantly reduced the salivary MS levels in the mothers. Fewer children colonized by MS in saliva compared with those in the control group. The treatment significantly reduced salivary MS levels in mothers and delayed bacterial colonization in their children for approximately 4 mo.

(continued on next page)

Table 1
(continued)

Author, Year, Country	Study Length, Design, and Objective	Sample Characteristics	Intervention	Clinical Outcomes		Results
				Mother	Child	
Zanata et al,[61] 2003, Brazil	Prospective 30-mo study to evaluate the effect of preventive measures taken in mother during pregnancy and caries experience in children for first time mothers	81 Mother-child pairs from pregnancy to 24 mo of age of child Divided into 2 groups: control and experimental	Both groups received an educational/primary preventive treatment. The experimental group also received 1. Primary care intervention composed of dental treatments 2. The topical application of NaF and iodine solution, carried out in 3 sessions: the first immediately after prophylaxis, and the second and third applications after 3 d and 5 d. The prophylactic measures were repeated during pregnancy and 6 mo and 12 mo after delivery. Both groups recalled every 6 mo; children also submitted for examination from 6 mo of age onward	PHP, CPITN, DMFS, and white spot lesions.	Caries in children—dmfs	A significant difference in caries prevalence was observed between children with and without visible dental plaque. The mean number of tooth surfaces with carious lesions (including areas of demineralization) was higher among the children in the control group compared with the experimental group however, with no statistical significance. Maternal caries increase was a significant factor influencing the caries experience of the children. These data support the evidence of an association between caries prevalence in young children and clinical (dental plaque) and maternal factors.

Motivational interviewing/counseling only

Harrison et al,[56] 2012, Canada	Cluster-randomized pragmatic (effectiveness) trial tested maternal counseling based on MI as an approach to control caries in indigenous children	241 Mother-child pairs For intervention: mothers who recently had given birth or were between the 12th wk and 34th wk of pregnancy were recruited For evaluation: children at 30 mo of age Mothers into 2 groups: test and control	Test group mothers were to attend 1 counseling session during pregnancy and up to 6 more sessions postnatally until their child's 2nd birthday. MI based on scripts from a previous trial (Weinstein et al,[80] 2004; Weinstein et al,[81] 2006): 1 script for pregnant and new mothers and another for those whose child had experienced the first tooth eruption. Mothers from test communities also received a Privilege Card to expedite dental care.	None	Enamel caries with substance loss	No statistically significant treatment effect was detected. Exploratory analyses suggested a substantial preventive effect for untreated decay at or beyond the level of the dentin and a particularly large treatment effect when mothers had 4 or more MI-style sessions. Overall, these results provide preliminary evidence that, for these young, indigenous children, an MI-style intervention has an impact on severity of caries

(continued on next page)

Table 1
(continued)

Author, Year, Country	Study Length, Design, and Objective	Sample Characteristics	Intervention	Clinical Outcomes Mother	Clinical Outcomes Child	Results
Plutzer & Spencer,[66] 2008, Australia Plutzer et al,[57] 2012	RCT to test the efficacy of an oral health promotion program for the parents of infants, starting during the pregnancy	649 women in 5th to 7th mo of pregnancy enrolled in the program (test group 327, control group 322); 441 had their child examined at follow-up.	Intervention group received 3 rounds of oral health promotion material: the first at their enrollment in the study and the other 2 by mail at 6 mo and 12 mo of child's age. After the 2nd round of information, the test group mothers were randomized again. The information was reinforced in 1 of the test subgroups through a telephone consultation. At 20 mo of age, children from both groups were examined by a dentist for the presence of any sign of ECC. Mothers were evaluated by total 4 questionnaires used during the study.	None	Earliest manifestation of S-ECC (US National Institute of Health definition)	The incidence of S-ECC in the test group was 1.7% and in the control group 9.6% (P < .001). An oral health promotion program based on repeated rounds of AG initiated during the mother's pregnancy on the prevention of ECC from before their child was born decreased the prevalence of ECC at 20 mo of age 5-fold.

Abbreviations: API, approximal plaque index; CPITN, community periodontal index of treatment needs; dft, decayed filled teeth-primary teeth; dmfs, decayed missing filled surface-primary teeth; DMFS, decayed missing filled surface-permanent teeth; DMFT, decayed missing filled teeth-permanent teeth; NaF, sodium fluoride; PHP, patient hygiene performance index; S, severe.

Table 2
Summary of intervention studies by type with mothers after childbirth up to 24 months to reduce mutans streptococci transmission and prevent caries in children (2000–2016)

Author, Year, and Country	Study Length, Design, and Objective	Sample Characteristics	Intervention	Clinical Outcomes		Results
				Mother	**Child**	
Xylitol						
Olak et al,[73] 2012, Finland	36-mo prospective study to compare the effect of xylitol usage among anxious and nonanxious mothers on caries experience in children	120 Mother-child pairs; recruited after birth of infants 60 YesX and 60 to NoX based on mother's choice Each group had 30 mothers from high level and low level of anxiety scores.	Intervention for 3 y All mothers screened for dental anxiety using Corah DAS and categorized into DAS high and DAS low. Baseline — at 3 mo of age of infants, both groups educated on oral hygiene and diet. At the end of baseline, questionnaire completed by mothers. YesX group: used xylitol lozenges (containing xylitol and maltitol [1:1]), 2 pieces 4×/ d (approximately: 5.8 g/d) until child 36 mo	Dental caries (WHO criteria) as DMFT at baseline	Dental caries (WHO criteria) examined twice at 2 and 3 y of age	Number of caries-free children were higher in xylitol-consuming group compared with control group at both 2 y and 3 y of age. No differences in proportion of caries in DAS high and low groups at both ages.

(continued on next page)

Table 2
(continued)

Author, Year, and Country	Study Length, Design, and Objective	Sample Characteristics	Intervention	Clinical Outcomes		Results
				Mother	Child	
Thorild et al,[70] 2004, Sweden Thorild et al,[71] 2006 Thorild et al,[72] 2012	3-y RCT (intervention — 1 y and outcomes at 3 y) To evaluate the effect of maternal use of chewing gums containing combinations of xylitol, sorbitol, CHX, and F on salivary (MS) counts and caries prevalence in children.	173 Mother-child pairs (6-mo-old infants, mothers with high MS) divided into 3 groups: 1. Xylitol (n = 61) 2. CHX + xylitol/ sorbitol (n = 55) 3. FX/sorbitol (n = 57)	Intervention for 1 y Started when the child was 6 mo old and terminated 1 y later. Mothers in different groups asked to chew gum for 5 min, 3 ×/d: xylitol: 650 mg xylitol/ piece — 3 pieces/d CHX + xylitol: 5 mg CHX + 533 mg xylitol/ piece — 3 pieces/d F + xylitol: 0.55 mg F + 289 mg xylitol/piece — 3 pieces/d	None	Salivary MS counts — Dentocult SM strip and caries (dft) at the age of 3 y.	At 3 y: lower but nonsignificant levels of salivary MS and dental decay were observed in 3-y-old children of mothers who used high-content xylitol gums.

| Fontana et al,[74] 2009, United States | 9-mo RCT to study the influence of xylitol gum on acquisition pattern of 39 bacterial species, including MS in infants. | High-risk mothers (MS levels ≥10^5 CFUs/mL of saliva) at the end of 3rd trimester or with infants <5 mo of age 97 mother-child pairs | Intervention for 9 mo Mothers divided into 4 groups: 1. Experimental: chewing xylitol gum (4.2 g/d), 2 pieces 3×/d after every meal for 5 min 2. Delayed experimental: mothers start chewing gum 6 mo after baseline examination for 9 mo same frequency as 1 3. Positive control: this group chewed xylitol gum the same frequency as the experimental group 4. Negative control: no chewing gum at all Mothers interviewed at baseline, 3 mo, 6 mo, and 9 mo of child's age. Dental examinations and MS sampled at baseline and at 9 mo for mother-child pair. | MS levels and DMFT (International Caries Detection and Assessment System criteria) and modified DMFT index for caries. | MS levels in infant and DNA profiles of different bacterial species. Selective culture: MSB for MS counts | Mothers' positive responses at baseline to "checking baby's food temperature by using baby's spoon" and "starting a bottle after stopping breast feeding" were significant predictors of MS counts in infants. No significant association between maternal xylitol and difference in microbial plaque composition for 9–14 mo old infants No significance between 39 different microbial species and different intervention groups |

(continued on next page)

Table 2
(continued)

Author, Year, and Country	Study Length, Design, and Objective	Sample Characteristics	Intervention	Clinical Outcomes		Results
				Mother	Child	
Söderling et al,[48] 2000, Finland Isokangas et al,[68] 2000 Söderling et al,[82] 2001 Laitala et al,[69] 2013	24-mo RCT to evaluate maternal use of xylitol chewing gum can prevent dental caries in their children by prohibiting the transmission of MS from mother to child	195 High-risk mothers (>10^5 CFUs/mL of saliva) and children (recruited at birth) into 3 groups: 1. Xylitol 2. CHX 3. FV Evaluation at 2 y of child's age with 169 mother-child pairs (106/ xylitol, 33/F, 30/ CHX).	Intervention for 21 mo Mothers were screened for high MS levels during pregnancy but interventions started after delivery. X group = chewing gum started 3 mo after delivery and discontinued 24 mo after the delivery The chewing gum xylitol as the only sweetener (65% xylitol), average daily dose of xylitol = 6–7 g, average 4×/d. CHX group = 3 CHX varnish (EC40) treatments. FV group = 3 FV (Duraphat); that is, 6 mo, 12 mo, and 18 mo after the delivery of the child All children of mothers of all groups regular examination; advice on diet, oral hygiene, and use of Fs, and, where necessary, restorative treatment	MS levels (2 mL of paraffin-stimulated whole saliva) at 6 mo, 12 mo, and 24 mo. Caries — DMFT (WHO) criteria) at 6 mo,	MS levels (pooled plaque samples) at 12 mo and 24 mo of age. Number of teeth present counted at 6 mo, 12 mo, and 24 mo of age	At 2 y old, the differences in MS levels were not significant between the FV and CHX groups. Fewer children in xylitol group had detectable levels of MS than children in other groups. At 3 y old, compared with the xylitol group, the risk of MS colonization was 2.3-fold higher in the FV group. The differences between the FV and CHX groups were significant. At 5 y old, dentinal caries (DMFT) in the xylitol group were reduced by 71% vs the FV group and 74% vs the CHX group. The difference between the CHX and FV group was not statistically significant.

Chlorhexidine — varnish

Gripp & Schlagenhauf,[75] 2002, Germany	24-mo RCT to study the influence of CHX varnish-mediated suppression of MS in mothers with high salivary MS counts on the frequency of MS colonization in their children at 2 y of age	44 Mother-child pairs. (children 20–137 d old at baseline). Divided into 3 groups based on MS levels. Group 1 CHX — high MS levels $\geq 10^5$ CFUs/mL of saliva; group 2 positive controls; and group 3 negative controls	Intervention for 24 mo All 3 groups were examined and educated with reinforcement of dietary habits and personal oral health habits. The CHX-intervention group also had preventive therapy and professional application of 40% CHX varnish every 3 mo.	MS levels: chairside test: Dentocult SM Strip in both groups every 3 mo, before and after session.	MS levels: selective culture: MSB every 6 mo until 24 mo of age	For mothers, a significant decrease in high MS values seen in the CHX group. For children at 24 mo, MS levels were significant in CHX and groups 2 and 3. The frequency of MS colonization in the CHX-treated group was not significantly different from the one found in a negative control group of 15 mother-child pairs with low maternal salivary MS levels.

(continued on next page)

Table 2
(continued)

Author, Year, and Country	Study Length, Design, and Objective	Sample Characteristics	Intervention	Clinical Outcomes		Results
				Mother	Child	
Dasanayake et al,[76] 2002, United States	24-mo RCT to study the effect of a 10% CHX varnish (Chlorzoin) on the mother-child transmission of MS and on subsequent caries experience	75 Mother-child pairs randomized into test and control groups: 1. CHX (n = 38) 2. Placebo varnish (n = 37) Mothers recruited when babies 6 mo old or approximately age of first tooth emergence	Intervention for 2 y Started with CHX/placebo applications first at 6 mo of babies age. Followed by 4 weekly applications of treatment/placebo varnish coinciding with the eruption of the first tooth. Subsequent to the first set of 4 applications, a single application was given every 6 mo, making the timing of application after the first set of 4 at 12 mo, 18 mo, 24 mo, 30 mo, and 36 mo after birth. Subjects were followed-up until the 4th birthday of the child. The treatment group received a 2-stage CHX varnish.	MS levels (stimulated saliva) and enamel and dentine caries: Pitts criteria 1994) and interproximal caries	MS levels: (pooled saliva and pooled plaque) Selective culture: MSB agar, Enamel and Dentine Caries: Pitts criteria 1994 and Interproximal caries	Mothers in the CHX group exhibited significantly low levels of MS levels in treatment group compared with 12 mo after the initial application. There were no significant differences in the percentage of children with detectable levels of S mutans in plaque during the study period. There were no significant differences in caries increment either among mothers or among children.

Preventive/restorative dental care and chlorhexidine rinse

| Ramos-Gomez et al,[77] 2011, United States | 2-y RCT to compare the efficacy of 2 prevention interventions in reducing ECC | 361 Mother-child dyads divided into intervention and control groups. Mothers were recruited during 2nd trimester of pregnancy. Interventions began 4 mo postpartum | Three interventions: 1. CHX mouth rinse for mother (rinse twice daily for 3 mo with 0.5-oz CHX on a 14-d rinse, 14-d rinse-free interval) 2. FV application in children 0.25 mL FV containing 5.6 mg F every 6 mo, from 12 mo to 36 mo 3. Parental oral health counseling. Control groups: (1) parental oral health counseling; (2) TherFV in children developing precavitated lesions. Intervention groups: (1) parental oral health counseling; (2) a 3-mo regimen of CHX mouth rinse for new mothers; (3) preventive FV applications for children | MS and LB levels (saliva samples at 3 mo prior to giving birth and with their children at 4 mo, 9 mo, 12 mo, 24 mo, and 36 mo postpartum) and caries (NIDCR caries diagnostic criteria) | MS and LB levels (saliva via spitting technique) and caries (NIDCR caries diagnostic criteria) | Parental counseling, a 3-mo maternal CHX regimen, and FV applied every 6 mo to children's teeth was not shown sufficient to significantly reduce caries and was not more efficacious than parental counseling alone combined with therapeutic FV for precavitated lesions. There was no significant difference in children's 36-month caries incidence between groups; 34% in each group developed caries. Maternal MS levels declined during CHX use but increased when discontinued. |

(continued on next page)

Table 2
(continued)

Author, Year, and Country	Study Length, Design, and Objective	Sample Characteristics	Intervention	Clinical Outcomes		Results
				Mother	Child	
Ercan et al,[78] 2007, Turkey	4-y Pilot study to evaluate the impact of preventive interventions in transmission of MS	8 Women (24–35 y of age) and their 11 children (2–11 mo of age) TMs = 8 TC = 11 TSb = 9 CC = 10	In the same tribe, mothers and their 11 children, and then (following years) their 9 siblings [TSb], were followed for 4 y. The study started when the teeth in TC group had just started to erupt. TMs were subjected to a preventive and restorative procedure. Also daily rinsing with 0.05% NaF during first 30 d, using 0.02% CHX rinses twice daily for 10 d in each 6-mo interval until the children are 3 y old was recommended. Examination of caries development and MS levels in TC and TSb were carried out annually and at 6-mo intervals. At the end of 4 y, 2 control groups: CC and Control Sibling resembling TC and TSb were selected from the other tribe living in the same village,	DMFT (WHO criteria for rural districts) MS levels: the modified-strip method —CRT Bacteria both at 6-mo and 12-mo	dmft index MS levels: children's plaque — the modified —strip method — CRT Bacteria both at 6 mo and 12 mo	Microbial data demonstrated that the TC and TSbs had significantly low bacterial level in plaque samples. They also had significantly low dmft and dmfs numbers compared with corresponding control group.

Motivational interviewing/counseling only

Weinstein et al,[80] 2004, Canada; Weinstein et al,[81] 2006; Harrison et al,[79] 2007	1-y RCT to compare the effect of MI counseling with traditional health education for mothers of young children at high risk of developing dental caries	240 Mother-child pairs; infants 6–18 mo of age enrolled in study. Randomized into 2 groups: 1. Test—MI 2. Control—traditional oral health education	Both groups received a pamphlet and viewed a video (11 min). Those in the MI group also received one 45-min MI counseling session at initial visit and 6 follow-up telephone calls during the 1st y to promote maintenance. Postcard reminders were also mailed in-between as reminders and reinforcers. There were no interventions in y 2. Each parent completed 2 interviews, assessing children's diet and other parental practices related to infant oral hygiene and feeding habits at bedtime.	None	Caries—dfs index, based on modification of Radike criteria	Evaluation at 1 y of age—children in MI group had 0.71 caries incidence compared with 1.91 in control group, which was statistically significant. Children in MI group had fewer new carious lesions compared with control group. Evaluation at 2 y: children in the MI group had 46% lower rate of DMFS at 2 y than the control group. Exploratory analysis revealed that rates of DMFS were higher in children whose mothers had prechewed their food, raised in rural environment, and higher family income.

Abbreviations: CC, control children; DAS, dental anxiety scale; dfs, decayed filled surface-mixed dentition; dft, decayed filled teeth-primary teeth; dmfs, decayed missing filled surface-primary teeth; DMFT, decayed missing filled teeth-permanent teeth; dmft, decayed missing filled teeth-primary teeth; F, fluoride; LB, lacto-bacilli; NaF, sodium fluoride; NIDCR, National Institute of Dental and Craniofacial Research; NoX, no xylitol group; TC, test children; TM, test mother; TherFV, therapeutic (rescue) FV; TSb, test sibling; WHO, world health organization; YesX, allocated to xylitol group.

mothers used CHX rinse for 3 months, and the intervention did not reduce caries in children.[77] One small pilot study reported reduced child MS and caries postintervention compared with controls.[78]

The MI intervention was effective in reducing caries prevalence and incidence in young children at follow-ups,[79–81] suggesting it is a promising preventive approach. The RCT compared MI (one 45-minute session plus 6 calls and postcards) to traditional education in high-risk South Asian immigrant mothers of 6-month-old to 18-month-old children in a nonfluoridated community in Canada. The MI counseling approach provides strategies to help individuals move to action and behavior change, as described by the stages of change theory.[83]

Effectiveness of the postdelivery maternal interventions was mixed. Across all the studies, child ages, intervention components, study length, and follow-up periods (ranged 9 months to 4 years), outcomes assessed and caries case definitions varied, which limit comparability across studies. Most study designs were robust; 7 interventions were RCTs and 1 was a prospective study, whereas 1 was a pilot study with a small sample size. More intervention studies of mother-infant pairs are needed to build the evidence base further in this area to inform which strategies are most effective for disrupting MS transmission and reducing caries in young children.

DISCUSSION

This is the first article to examine maternal intervention effectiveness on MS reductions and child caries for young children under 24 months by pregnancy status. Consistent findings suggest AG and MI are important during the prenatal and postdelivery periods. Evidence was more supportive of prenatal clinical interventions yielding intended reductions on MS levels and caries in children. Postdelivery evidence was more mixed, but many interventions included multiple components, with some interventions also targeting the young child.

Recent reviews focused on just xylitol interventions and concluded the evidence did not support that xylitol use consistently reduced MS or caries in children.[84,85] Those reviews, however, had broader inclusion criteria. Some studies reviewed focused on interventions with older children and adults, and results were mixed. Two other narrower reviews concluded habitual use of xylitol gums and other polyols to be effective in reducing transmission and caries in children when used prenatally or after delivery by mothers.[86,87] A meta-analysis of 41 studies from 1998 to 2014 focused on the impact of antimicrobial interventions on ECC. Li and Tanner[87] concluded that temporary MS reductions were found, but longer-term impact was questionable. There is a call for more robust research to drive clinical guidelines in this area.[88]

Dental Care for Pregnant Women

In 2012, the Oral Health Care During Pregnancy national workgroup released a major consensus statement reinforcing the need to provide dental care to expectant mothers and not delay treatment, which is safe in any trimester.[54] Yet, misconceptions about the safety and effectiveness of providing dental care remain, and dentists lack training about current evidence for treating pregnant women.[89] The American Congress of Obstetricians and Gynecologists recommends a dental screening at the first prenatal visit to increase the likelihood of early intervention.[90] The importance of good oral health of both mother and child is consistently outlined, including oral hygiene and dental care utilization practices. Establishing a healthy oral environment is important for pregnant women and can be achieved at home with adequate plaque control, such as brushing, flossing, and use of fluoridated toothpaste and antimicrobial agents, such as xylitol and CHX rinses. This can be followed by a professional prophylaxis, including coronal scaling, root planning, and polishing.[91] These practices should be maintained after childbirth to promote oral health for both mother and infant.

Six-Step Infant Oral Care Protocol

Establishing a dental home is critical for ECC prevention in earliest childhood. Mothers who use dental care regularly are more likely to take their child to a dentist.[92] Primary caregivers also influence the age at which a child first seeks dental care.[93] An infant's first dental visit is recommended at first tooth eruption or age 1,[94] although this does not occur for most.[11] The Caries Management by Risk Assessment (CAMBRA) tool and approach integrates risk assessment of childhood caries in a comprehensive oral health visit to promote good oral health for infants and new mothers.

The 6-step protocol,[95] a simple and systematic method to effectively conduct preventive infant oral visits, consists of the following:

1. Caries risk assessment using the CAMBRA tool[96] (**Fig. 2**)
   - CAMBRA assists providers to systematically assess each child and his/her caregiver's caries risk in an individualized manner that tailors a specific preventive therapeutic management plan for the family, using a disease management protocol (**Table 3**).
2. Proper knee-to-knee positioning of a child
   - This allows for effective and efficient visualization of a child's dentition.
3. Age-appropriate toothbrushing prophylaxis
   - This step is an effective way of removing plaque on most teeth and should be conducted using fluoridated toothpaste appropriate to a child's age. Children ages 0 to 3 are recommended to use a smear of toothpaste or the size of a grain of rice.[94]
4. Clinical examination of a child's oral cavity and dentition
5. Fluoride varnish (FV) treatment
   - FV application every 3 months to 6 months prevents tooth decay, depending on a child's caries risk
6. AG, counseling, and establishment of self-management goals (**Fig. 3**)
   - Establishing 2 family-appropriate self-management goals should be a mutual decision between the parent and provider, encouraging families to adopt a healthy oral lifestyle.

The age 2 infant oral care visit introduces children to routine care that is the foundation to their lifelong oral health and physical well-being. A growing body of evidence supports that an early oral health intervention program, consisting of caries risk assessment, clinical examination, and a treatment plan based on a child's caries risk level, is efficacious in ECC prevention.[97] Preventive therapies should drive clinical caries management in young children, with restorative care only provided as needed.[98] The American Academy of Pediatrics updated their preventive oral health care recommendations in October 2015, adding an FV subheading specifically and indicating its use for children from 6 months to age 5.[99] Pediatric well-child visits should also include oral health screenings and AG routinely and dentist referral if needed. Pediatricians frequently see young children within the first 24 months of life. Community-based infant oral care programs should also address maternal oral health[100] and provide culturally appropriate education based on risk level and account for variations in health literacy.

CARIES RISK ASSESSMENT FORM FOR AGES 0 TO 5 YRS OLD

Patient Name: _____ I.D. #_____ Age: _____

Date: _____ Assessment Date: _____

NOTE: Any one YES in Column 1 signifies likely "High Risk" and an indication for bacteria tests	YES = CIRCLE			Comments:
	1	2	3	
1. Risk Factors (Biological Predisposing Factors)				
(a) Mother/caregiver has active dental decay in past year	YES			
(b) Bottle with fluid other than water, plain milk and/or formula		YES		Type(s):
(c) Continual bottle use		YES		
(d) Child sleeps with a bottle, or nurses on demand		YES		
(e) Frequent (> 3 times/day) between-meal snacks of sugars/cooked starch/sugared beverages		YES		# times/day: Type(s):
(f) Saliva-Reducing factors are present, including: 1. medications (e.g., asthma [albuterol] or hyperactivity) 2. medical (cancer treatment) or genetic factors		YES		
(g) Child has Special Health Care Needs		YES		
(h) Parent and/or caregiver has low SES (Socio-economic status) and/or low health literacy, WIC/Early Head Start		YES		
2. Protective Factors				
(a) Child lives in a fluoridated community (note zip code)			YES	Zip Code:
(b) Takes fluoride supplements			YES	
(c) Child drinks fluoridated water (e.g., tap water)			YES	
(d) Teeth brushed with fluoride toothpaste (pea size) at least 2x daily			YES	# times/day:
(e) Fluoride varnish in last 6 months			YES	
(f) Mother/caregiver understands use of xylitol gum/lozenges			YES	
(g) Child is given xylitol (recommended wipes, spray, gel)			YES	
3. Disease Indicators - Clinical Examination of Child				
(a) Obvious white spots, decalcifications, or decay present on the child's teeth	YES			
(b) Existing restorations	YES			
(c) Plaque is obvious on the teeth and/or gums bleed easily		YES		
(d) Visually inadequate saliva flow		YES		
(e) New remineralization since last visit (List teeth):			YES	Teeth:

Child's Overall Caries Risk (circle):   HIGH   MODERATE   LOW

Child: Bacteria/Saliva Test Results: MS: LB: Flow Rate: ml/min: Date:
Caregiver: Bacteria/Saliva Test Results: MS: LB: Flow Rate: ml/min: Date:

Self-management goals:

1. _____

2. _____

Clinician's Signature: _____

Since Last Visit:

New Cavitation: Y / N
New White Spot Lesions: Y / N
Dental Pain: Y / N
Referral Type: O.R.   I.V.   Oral Sedation
Date: _____   (Updated: 5/1/14)

Fig. 2. CAMBRA form. (*Reprinted with permission from* the California Dental Association, copyright October 2011.)

PROMISING STRATEGIES

Future intervention efforts should continue to build on existing clinical evidence and always include patient education to promote prevention for mother and infant. Pregnancy is a teachable moment; expectant mothers are inclined to improve health behaviors for themselves and an unborn child. New motherhood is also a prime time for education. First-time mothers in particular may be overwhelmed with the transition to motherhood but are usually interested in providing optimal care and reducing health risks for themselves and their newborns and infants. Education is necessary but never sufficient for sustained behavior change.[101] Prenatal health education should include information about ECC etiology and prevention, emphasizing infant feeding and hygiene instruction, the age 1 first dental visit, and recommendations for maintaining optimal maternal oral health during pregnancy and after childbirth to reduce MS transmission.

Table 3
Example of a caries management protocol for 0–2 year olds

| Risk Category Ages 0–2 | Diagnostic | | | Preventive Intervention | | | | | | | Restoration |
	Periodic Oral Examinations	Radiographs	Saliva Test	Fluoride	Xylitol	Sealants	Antibacterials/ Probiotics	Anticipatory Guidance/ Counseling	Self-management Goals	White Spot/ Precavitated Lesions	Existing Lesions
Low	Annual	Posterior bitewings at 12–24 mo intervals if proximal surfaces cannot be examined visually or with a probe	Optional baseline	In office: no home: brush 2×/d with smear of F toothpaste	Not Required	No	No	Yes	No	N/A	N/A
Moderate	Every 6 mo	Posterior bitewings at 6–12 mo intervals if proximal surfaces cannot be examined visually or with a probe	Suggested	In office: FV initial visit and recalls Home: brush 2×/d with smear of F toothpaste Caregiver: OTC NaF treatment rinses	Child: xylitol wipes 3×–4× daily Caregiver: 2 sticks of gum or 2 mints 4×/d, total 6–10 g/d	Glass ionomer–based materials recommended on deep pits and fissures	No	Yes	No	Treat with F products as indicated to promote remineralization	N/A

(continued on next page)

Table 3
(continued)

Risk Category Ages 0-2	Diagnostic			Preventive Intervention						Restoration	
	Periodic Oral Examinations	Radiographs	Saliva Test	Fluoride	Xylitol	Sealants	Antibacterials/ Probiotics	Anticipatory Guidance/ Counseling	Self-management Goals	White Spot/ Precavitated Lesions	Existing Lesions
Moderate; noncompliant	Every 3–6 mo	Posterior bitewings at 6–12 mo intervals if proximal surfaces cannot be examined visually or with a probe	Recommended	In office: FV initial visit and recalls Home: brush 2×/d with smear of F toothpaste then apply a smear of calcium phosphate paste left on at bedtime Caregiver: OTC NaF treatment rinses	Child: xylitol wipes 3×– 4× daily Caregiver: 2 sticks of gum or 2 mints 4×/d, total 6–10 g/d	Glass ionomer-based materials recommended on deep pits and fissures	Recommend CHX for caregiver/ recommend probiotics	Yes	Yes	Treat with F products as indicated to promote remineralization	N/A

High	Every 3 mo	Anterior (#2 occlusal film) and posterior bitewings at 6–12 mo intervals if proximal surfaces cannot be examined visually or with a probe	Recom-mended	In office: FV initial visit and recalls Home: brush 2×/d with smear of F toothpaste then apply a smear of calcium phosphate paste left on at bedtime Caregiver: OTC NaF treatment rinses	Child: Xylitol wipes 3×–4× daily Caregiver: 2 sticks of gum or 2 mints 4×/d, total 6–10 g/d	Glass ionomer–based materials recommended on deep pits and fissures	Recommend CHX for caregiver/recommend probiotics	Yes	Yes	Treat with F products as indicated to promote remineralization	ITRs with glass ionomer–based materials or conventional restorative treatment as patient cooperation and family circumstances allow
High; noncompliant	Every 1–3 mo	Anterior (#2 occlusal film) and posterior bitewings at 6–12 mo intervals if proximal surfaces cannot be examined visually or with a probe	Recom-mended	In office: FV initial visit and recalls Home: brush 2×/d with smear of F toothpaste then apply a smear of calcium phosphate paste left on at bedtime Caregiver: OTC NaF treatment rinses	Child: xylitol wipes 3×–4× daily Caregiver: 2 sticks of gum or 2 mints 4×/d, total 6–10 g/d	Glass ionomer–based materials recommended on deep pits and fissures	Recommend CHX for caregiver/recommend probiotics	Yes	Yes	Treat with F products as indicated to promote remineralization	ITRs with glass ionomer–based materials or conventional restorative treatment as patient cooperation and family circumstances allow

(continued on next page)

**Table 3
(continued)**

Risk Category Ages 0–2	Diagnostic			Preventive Intervention						Restoration	
	Periodic Oral Examinations	Radiographs	Saliva Test	Fluoride	Xylitol	Sealants	Antibacterials/ Probiotics	Anticipatory Guidance/ Counseling	Self-management Goals	White Spot/ Precavitated Lesions	Existing Lesions
Extreme	Every 1–3 mo	Anterior (#2 occlusal film) and posterior bitewings at 6–12 mo intervals if proximal surfaces cannot be examined visually or with a probe	Recommended	In office: FV initial visit and recalls Home: brush 2×/d with smear of F toothpaste then apply a smear of calcium phosphate paste left on at bedtime Caregiver: OTC NaF treatment rinses	Child: xylitol wipes 3×– 4× daily Caregiver: 2 sticks of gum or 2 mints 4×/d, total 6–10 g/d	Glass ionomer–based materials recommended on deep pits and fissures	Recommend CHX for caregiver/ recommend probiotics	Yes	Yes	Treat with F products as indicated to promote remineralization	ITRs with glass ionomer–based materials or conventional restorative treatment as patient coperation and family circumstances allow

Abbreviations: CHX, chlorhexidine; F, fluoride; FV, fluoride varnish; ITR, interim therapeutic restoration; NaF, sodium fluoride; OTC, over the counter.

Courtesy of the California Dental Association; with permission.

Patient Name   DOB

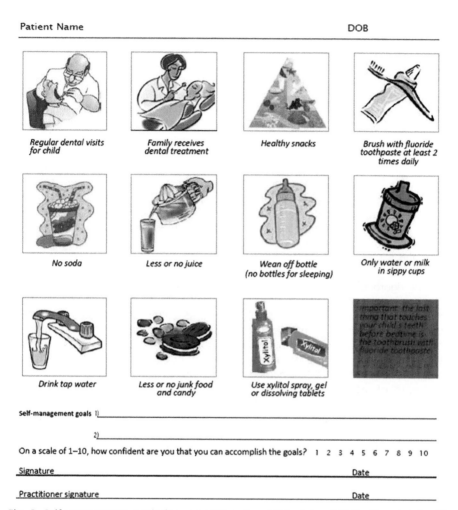

Fig. 3. Self-management goals for parent/caregiver. DOB, date of birth. (*Reprinted with permission from* the California Dental Association, copyright October 2011.)

MI is a promising patient-centered counseling technique used in ECC prevention intervention studies for motivating caregiver behavior change. This review found positive evidence for MI starting in pregnancy and postdelivery on ECC outcomes, although this is only based on 3 studies. None of the MI studies assessed maternal oral health or included other intervention components like antimicrobials, and these could be useful additions to test in future interventions. A recent systematic review included 5 postdelivery dental studies, also suggesting MI can improve caregivers' preventive behaviors and child ECC outcomes.[102] An RCT 4-part intervention study comparing MI, AG, and dental care during pregnancy versus a delayed group (receiving the intervention postpartum) is under way in Australia; results will inform the effectiveness of these strategies during pregnancy.[103]

FUTURE RESEARCH DIRECTIONS

Scant data are available in the United States to support conducting research in this area. The Pregnancy Risk Assessment Monitoring System survey includes 5 dental utilization/barriers questions, but not all are pregnancy-specific.[104] NHANES includes pregnancy status, oral health survey measures, and clinical dental examinations. Neither data set follows a cohort longitudinally. Long-term intergenerational considerations have not been extensively studied in oral health yet would be valuable data to collect to help advance the field.[105] Interdisciplinary approaches to address multiple determinants of ECC for mothers and infants are also needed.[106]

Data on pregnant and postpartum women's oral hygiene behaviors and clinically assessed oral health status, including salivary indicators, is also scarce. Pregnancy is often an exclusionary criterion in research, unless it is part of a study's central purpose. More longitudinal studies are needed to follow pregnant women during pregnancy and for the first 2 or more years postdelivery, especially in high-risk populations. Collecting clinical, biological, and validated survey measures together from mother-infant dyads will yield richer data, enabling in-depth analysis and exploration of prenatal risk factors and effective early interventions for MS reduction and ECC prevention. A US-based study, the Centering Pregnancy Oral Health Promotion Extension, is currently testing an oral health promotion intervention in a prenatal program and will compare salivary bacteria of infants at 6 months and 12 months of age.[107]

More rigorously designed RCT studies with appropriate control groups and placebos for promising antimicrobials like xylitol should be conducted with pregnant women and mothers of infants and toddlers to study their impact on mothers and young children and long-term effectiveness.[88] Studies designed to test the efficacy and effectiveness, account for potentially confounding variables, and assess mediating or moderating factors are needed and may not all be answerable in a single study. If interventions are multicomponent, this complicates interpreting the fidelity and impact of each component as a preventive agent and if it is truly clinically beneficial. Results also need replicating with other samples, to examine acceptability and feasibility with different population groups. None of the studies reviewed in this article included cost, but cost-effectiveness may need to be considered in the future and affect clinical recommendations. More long-term studies are needed that start during pregnancy or soon after childbirth, and they should continue to examine the extent of mother and child MS reduction and linkage to young children's caries outcomes.

SUMMARY

A growing body of evidence from maternal interventions during pregnancy and post-delivery support that early prenatal interventions are effective at reducing mother-child MS transmission and delay MS colonization and caries in children. Dental care during pregnancy is safe, effective, and recommended. Dental screenings and AG about maternal and infant oral health should be part of regular prenatal care. Maternal interventions postdelivery help reduce MS transmission. Early infant oral care following a simple, systematic 6-step visit protocol, including caries risk assessment, is also recommended for addressing maternal behavioral risk factors, setting self-management goals, and promoting optimal oral health for the whole family.

REFERENCES

1. Laine MA. Effect of pregnancy on periodontal and dental health. Acta Odontol Scand 2002;60(5):257–64.
2. Löe H. Periodontal changes in pregnancy. J Periodontol 1965;36:209–17.
3. Wu M, Chen S-W, Jiang S-Y. Relationship between gingival inflammation and pregnancy. Mediators Inflamm 2015;2015:623427.

4. Niederman R. Pregnancy gingivitis and causal inference. Evid Based Dent 2013;14(4):107–8.
5. Steinberg BJ, Hilton IV, Iida H, et al. Oral health and dental care during pregnancy. Dent Clin North Am 2013;57(2):195–210.
6. Drury TF, Horowitz AM, Ismail AI, et al. Diagnosing and reporting early childhood caries for research purposes. J Public Health Dent 1999;59(3):192–7.
7. Dye BA, Hsu K-LC, Afful J. Prevalence and measurement of dental caries in young children. Pediatr Dent 2015;37(3):200–16.
8. Eckert GJ, Jackson R, Fontana M. Sociodemographic variation of caries risk factors in toddlers and caregivers. Int J Dent 2010;2010.
9. Fisher-Owens SA, Gansky SA, Platt LJ, et al. Influences on children's oral health: a conceptual model. Pediatr 2007;120(3):e510–20.
10. Harris R, Nicoll AD, Adair PM, et al. Risk factors for dental caries in young children: a systematic review of the literature. Community Dent Health 2004; 21(Suppl 1):71–85.
11. Gussy MG, Waters EG, Walsh O, et al. Early childhood caries: current evidence for aetiology and prevention. J Paediatr Child Health 2006;42(1–2):37.
12. Leong PM, Gussy MG, Barrow S-YL, et al. A systematic review of risk factors during first year of life for early childhood caries. Int J Paediatr Dent 2013; 23(4):235–50.
13. Hooley M, Skouteris H, Boganin C, et al. Parental influence and the development of dental caries in children aged 0–6 years: a systematic review of the literature. J Dent 2012;40(11):873–85.
14. Mattos-Graner RO, Klein MI, Smith DJ. Lessons learned from clinical studies: roles of mutans streptococci in the pathogenesis of dental caries. Curr Oral Health Rep 2014;1(1):70–8.
15. Law V, Seow WK, Townsend G. Factors influencing oral colonization of mutans streptococci in young children. Aust Dent J 2007;52(2):93–100.
16. Martinez G, Daniels K, Chandra A. Fertility of men and women aged 15-44 years in the United States: National Survey of Familiy Growth, 2006–2010. Hyattsville, MD: National Health Statistics Report; 2012.
17. Hamilton BE, Martin JA, Osterman MJ, et al. Births: final data for 2014. Natl Vita Stat Rep 2015;64(12):1–64.
18. Mathews TJ, Hamilton BE. Mean age of mothers is on the rise: United States, 2000–2014. Hyattsville (MD): National Center for Health Statistics; 2016.
19. State Adolescent Health Resources Center. Developmental tasks and attributes of late adolescence/young adulthood (ages 18-24 years). Konopka Institute, University of Minnesota. Available at: http://www.amchp.org/programsandtopics/ AdolescentHealth/projects/Documents/SAHRC%20AYADevelopment%20Late AdolescentYoungAdulthood.pdf. Accessed September 30, 2016.
20. American Academy of Pediatric Dentistry Committee on Clinical Affairs, Committee on the Adolescent. Guideline on oral health care for the pregnant adolescent. Pediatr Dent 2012;34(5):153–9.
21. Chaffee BW, Gansky SA, Weintraub JA, et al. Maternal oral bacterial levels predict Early Childhood Caries development. J Dent Res 2014;93(3):238–44.
22. Boggess KA, Urlaub DM, Massey KE. Oral hygiene practices and dental service utilization among pregnant women. J Am Dent Assoc 2010;141(5):553–61.
23. Timothé P, Eke PI, Presson SM, et al. Dental care use among pregnant women in the United States Reported in 1999 and 2002. Prev Chronic Dis 2005;2(1):A10.

24. Gaffield ML, Gilbert BJ, Malvitz DM, et al. Oral health during pregnancy: an analysis of information collected by the pregnancy risk assessment monitoring system. J Am Dent Assoc 2001;132(7):1009–16.

25. Lydon-Rochelle MT, Krakowiak P, Hujoel PP, et al. Dental care use and self-reported dental problems in relation to pregnancy. Am J Public Health 2004; 94(5):765–71.

26. Hwang S, Smith V, McCormick M, et al. Racial/ethnic disparities in maternal oral health experiences in 10 states, pregnancy risk assessment monitoring system, 2004–2006. Matern Child Health J 2011;15(6):722–9.

27. Needleman HL, Allred E, Bellinger D, et al. Antecedents and correlates of hypoplastic enamel defects of primary incisors. Pediatr Dent 1991;14(3):158–66.

28. Jacobsen PE, Haubek D, Henriksen TB, et al. Developmental enamel defects in children born preterm: a systematic review. Eur J Oral Sci 2014;122(1):7–14.

29. Julihn A, Ekbom A, Modéer T. Maternal overweight and smoking: prenatal risk factors for caries development in offspring during the teenage period. Eur J Epidemiol 2009;24(12):753–62.

30. Chung LH, Gregorich SE, Armitage GC, et al. Sociodemographic disparities and behavioral factors in clinical oral health status during pregnancy. Community Dent Oral Epidemiol 2014;42(2):151–9.

31. Weintraub JA, Finlayson TL, Gansky SA, et al. Clinically determined and self-reported dental status during and after pregnancy among low-income Hispanic women. J Public Health Dent 2013;73(4):311–20.

32. Azofeifa A, Yeung LF, Alverson CJ, et al. Dental caries and periodontal disease among U.S. pregnant women and nonpregnant women of reproductive age, National Health and Nutrition Examination Survey, 1999–2004. J Public Health Dent 2016;76(4):320–9.

33. Abreu LG, Elyasi M, Badri P, et al. Factors associated with the development of dental caries in children and adolescents in studies employing the life course approach: a systematic review. Eur J Oral Sci 2015;123(5):305–11.

34. Reisine S, Litt M, Tinanoff N. A biopsychosocial model to predict caries in preschool children. Pediatr Dent 1994;16(6):413–8.

35. Finlayson TL, Siefert K, Ismail AI, et al. Psychosocial factors and early childhood caries among low-income African-American children in Detroit. Community Dent Oral Epidemiol 2007;35(6):439–48.

36. Lapirattanakul J, Nakano K. Mother-to-child transmission of mutans streptococci. Future Microbiol 2014;9(6):807–23.

37. Kohler B, Andreen I, Jonsson B. The effect of caries-preventive measures in mothers on dental caries and the oral presence of the bacteria Streptococcus mutans and lactobacilli in their children. Arch Oral Biol 1984;29(11):879–83.

38. Li Y, Caufield PW. The fidelity of initial acquisition of mutans streptococci by infants from their mothers. J Dent Res 1995;74(2):681–5.

39. Berkowitz RJ. Mutans streptococci: acquisition and transmission. Pediatr Dent 2006;28(2):106–9 [discussion: 192–8].

40. Tanzer JM, Livingston J, Thompson AM. The microbiology of primary dental caries in humans. J Dent Educ 2001;65(10):1028–37.

41. Thorild I, Lindau-jonson B, Twetman S. Prevalence of salivary Streptococcus mutans in mothers and in their preschool children. Int J Paediatr Dent 2002; 12(1):2–7.

42. Douglass JM, Li Y, Tinanoff N. Association of Mutans Streptococci between caregivers and their children. Pediatr Dent 2008;30(5):375–87.

43. Wan AK, Seow WK, Purdie DM, et al. Oral colonization of Streptococcus mutans in six-month-old predentate infants. J Dent Res 2001;80(12):2060–5.
44. Wan AK, Seow WK, Walsh LJ, et al. Association of Streptococcus mutans infection and oral developmental nodules in pre-dentate infants. J Dent Res 2001; 80(10):1945–8.
45. Caufield PW, Cutter GR, Dasanayake AP. Initial acquisition of mutans Streptococci by infants: evidence for a discrete window of infectivity. J Dental Res 1993;72(1):37–45.
46. Alaluusua S, Renkonen OV. Streptococcus mutans establishment and dental caries experience in children from 2 to 4 years old. Scand J Dent Res 1983; 91(6):453–7.
47. Kohler B, Andreen I, Jonsson B. The earlier the colonization by mutans streptococci, the higher the caries prevalence at 4 years of age. Oral Microbiol Immunol 1988;3(1):14–7.
48. Söderling E, Isokangas P, Pienihäkkinen K, et al. Influence of maternal xylitol consumption on acquisition of Mutans Streptococci by infants. J Dental Res 2000;79(3):882–7.
49. Alaluusua S. Streptococcus mutans establishment and changes in salivary IgA in young children with reference to dental caries. Longitudinal studies and studies on associated methods. Proc Finn Dent Soc 1983;79(Suppl 3):1–55.
50. Thomson WM, Poulton R, Milne BJ, et al. Socioeconomic inequalities in oral health in childhood and adulthood in a birth cohort. Community Dent Oral Epidemiol 2004;32(5):345–53.
51. Köhler B, Andréen I. Mutans Streptococci and caries prevalence in children after early maternal caries prevention: a follow-up at 19 years of age. Caries Res 2012;46(5):474–80.
52. Richards D, Duane B, Sherriff A. Maternal consumption of xylitol for preventing dental decay in children. Cochrane Database Syst Rev 2012;(11):CD010202.
53. Riggs E, Slack-Smith L, Yelland J, et al. Interventions with pregnant women and new mothers for preventing caries in children (protocol). Cochrane Database Syst Rev 2016;(4):CD012155.
54. Oral Health Care During Pregnancy Expert Workgroup. Oral health care during pregnancy: a national consensus statement - Summary of an Expert Workgroup Meeting. Washington, DC: National Maternal and Child Oral Health Resource Center; 2012.
55. Milgrom P, Ly KA, Roberts MC. Mutans Streptococci dose response to xylitol chewing gum. J Dent Res 2006;85(2):177–81.
56. Harrison RL, Veronneau J, Leroux B. Effectiveness of maternal counseling in reducing caries in Cree children. J Dent Res 2012;91(11):1032–7.
57. Plutzer K, Spencer AJ, Keirse MJNC. Reassessment at 6–7years of age of a randomized controlled trial initiated before birth to prevent early childhood caries. Community Dent Oral Epidemiol 2012;40(2):116–24.
58. Shinga-Ishihara C, Nakai Y, Milgrom P, et al. Xylitol carryover effects on salivary Mutans Streptococci after 13 months of chewing xylitol gum. Caries Res 2012; 46(6):519–22.
59. Gomez SS, Weber AA. Effectiveness of a caries preventive program in pregnant women and new mothers on their offspring. Int J Paediatr Dent 2001;11(2): 117–22.
60. Nakai Y, Shinga-Ishihara C, Kaji M, et al. Xylitol gum and maternal transmission of mutans streptococci. J Dent Res 2010;89(1):56–60.

61. Zanata RL, Navarro MF, Pereira JC, et al. Effect of caries preventive measures directed to expectant mothers on caries experience in their children. Brazil Dent J 2003;14:75–81.

62. Günay H, Dmoch-Bockhorn K, Gunay Y, et al. Effect on caries experience of a long-term preventive program for mothers and children starting during pregnancy. Clin Oral Investig 1998;2(3):137–42.

63. Meyer K, Geurtsen W, Günay H. An early oral health care program starting during pregnancy. Clin Oral Investig 2010;14(3):257–64.

64. Meyer K, Khorshidi-Böhm M, Geurtsen W, et al. An early oral health care program starting during pregnancy—a long-term study—phase V. Clin Oral Investig 2014;18(3):863–72.

65. Brambilla E, Felloni A, Gagliani M, et al. Caries prevention during pregnancy: Results of a 30-month study. J Am Dent Assoc 1998;129(7):871–7.

66. Plutzer K, Spencer AJ. Efficacy of an oral health promotion intervention in the prevention of early childhood caries. Community Dent Oral Epidemiol 2008; 36(4):335–46.

67. Gomez SS, Weber AA, Emilson C-G. A prospective study of a caries prevention program in pregnant women and their children five and six years of age. ASDC J Dent Child 2001;68(3):191–5.

68. Isokangas P, Soderling E, Pienihakkinen K, et al. Occurrence of dental decay in children after maternal consumption of xylitol chewing gum, a follow-up from 0 to 5 years of age. J Dental Res 2000;79(11):1885–9.

69. Laitala ML, Alanen P, Isokangas P, et al. Long-term effects of maternal prevention on children's dental decay and need for restorative treatment. Community Dent Oral Epidemiol 2013;41(6):534–40.

70. Thorild I, Lindau B, Twetman S. Salivary mutans streptococci and dental caries in three-year-old children after maternal exposure to chewing gums containing combinations of xylitol, sorbitol, chlorhexidine, and fluoride. Acta Odontol Scand 2004;62(5):245–50.

71. Thorild I, Lindau B, Twetman S. Caries in 4-year old children after maternal chewing of gums containing combinations of xylitol, sorbitol, chlorhexidine and fluoride. Eur Arch Paediatr Dent 2006;7(4):241–5.

72. Thorild I, Lindau B, Twetman S. Long-term effect of maternal xylitol exposure on their children's caries prevalence. Eur Arch Paediatr Dent 2012;13(6):305–7.

73. Olak J, Saag M, Vahlberg T, et al. Caries prevention with xylitol lozenges in children related to maternal anxiety. A demonstration project. Eur Arch Paediatr Dent 2012;13(2):64–9.

74. Fontana M, Catt D, Eckert GJ, et al. Xylitol: effects on the acquisition of cariogenic species in infants. Pediatr Dent 2009;31(3):257–66.

75. Gripp VC, Schlagenhauf U. Prevention of early Mutans Streptococci transmission in infants by professional tooth cleaning and chlorhexidine varnish treatment of the mother. Caries Res 2002;36(5):366–72.

76. Dasanayake AP, Li Y, Wadhawan S, et al. Disparities in dental service utilization among Alabama Medicaid children. Community Dent Oral Epidemiol 2002; 30(5):369–76.

77. Ramos-Gomez FJ, Gansky SA, Featherstone JDB, et al. Mother and youth access (MAYA) maternal chlorhexidine, counselling and paediatric fluoride varnish randomized clinical trial to prevent early childhood caries. Int J Paediatr Dent 2011;22(3):169–79.

78. Ercan E, Dülgergil ÇT, Yildirim I, et al. Prevention of maternal bacterial transmission on children's dental-caries-development: 4-year results of a pilot study in a rural-child population. Arch Oral Biol 2007;52(8):748–52.
79. Harrison R, Benton T, Everson-Stewart S, et al. Effect of motivational interviewing on rates of early childhood caries: a randomized trial. Pediatr Dent 2007;29(1): 16–22.
80. Weinstein P, Harrison R, Benton T. Motivating parents to prevent caries in their young children: one-year findings. J Am Dent Assoc 2004;135(6):731–8.
81. Weinstein P, Harrison R, Benton T. Motivating mothers to prevent caries: confirming the beneficial effect of counseling. J Am Dent Assoc 2006;137(6):789–93.
82. Söderling E, Isokangas P, Pienihäkkinen K, et al. Influence of maternal xylitol consumption on mother–child transmission of Mutans Streptococci: 6–year follow–up. Caries Res 2001;35(3):173–7.
83. DiClemente CC, Velasquez MM. Motivational interviewing and the stages of change. In: Motivational interviewing: preparing people for change. 2002;2:201–16.
84. American Academy of Pediatric Dentistry Council on Clinical Affairs. Policy on the use of xylitol. Pediatr Dent 2016;38(6):47–9.
85. Riley P, Moore D, Sharif MO, et al. Xylitol-containing products for preventing dental caries in children and adults. Cochrane Database Syst Rev 2015;(3):CD010743.
86. Milgrom P, Söderling EM, Nelson S, et al. Clinical evidence for polyol efficacy. Adv Dent Res 2012;24(2):112–6.
87. Li Y, Tanner A. Effect of Antimicrobial Interventions on the Oral Microbiota Associated with Early Childhood Caries. Pediatr Dent 2015;37(3):226–44.
88. Fontana M, González-Cabezas C. Are we ready for definitive clinical guidelines on xylitolp/polyol use? Adv Dent Res 2012;24(2):123–8.
89. Vieira DR, de Oliveira AE, Lopes FF, et al. Dentists' knowledge of oral health during pregnancy: a review of the last 10 years' publications. Community Dent Health 2015;32(2):77–82.
90. American College of Obstetricians and Gynecologists Women's Health Care Physicians, Committee on Health Care for Underserved WomenAmerican Congress of Obstetricians and Gynecologists. Committee opinion no. 569: oral health care during pregnancy and through the lifespan. Obstet Gynecol 2013;122(2 PART 1):417–22.
91. California Dental Association Foundation. Oral health during pregnancy and early childhood: evidence-based guidelines for health professionals. Executive Summary. 2010. Available at: http://www.cdafoundation.org/Portals/0/pdfs/poh_guidelines.pdf. Accessed December 20, 2016.
92. Grembowski D, Spiekerman C, Milgrom P. Linking mother and child access to dental care. Pediatr 2008;122(4):e805–14.
93. Divaris K, Lee JY, Baker AD, et al. Influence of caregivers and children's entry into the dental care system. Pediatr 2014;133(5):e1268–76.
94. American Academy of Pediatric Dentistry Council on Clinical Affairs. Guideline on Caries-risk assessment and management for infants, children, and adolescents. Pediatr Dent 2016;38(6):142–9.
95. Ramos-Gomez F, Ng M-W. Into the future: keeping healthy teeth caries free: pediatric CAMBRA protocols. J Calif Dent Assoc 2011;39(10):723–33.
96. Ramos-Gomez F, Crall JJ, Gansky SA, et al. Caries risk assessment appropriate for the age 1 visit (infants and toddlers). J Calif Dent Assoc 2007;35(10): 687–702.

97. Ramos-Gomez F, Ng MW. Six step protocol for a successful infant oral care visit. Pediatr Dent Today 2009;38–40.

98. Slayton RL. Clinical decision-making for caries management in children: An update. Pediatr Dent 2015;37(2):106–10.

99. Committee on practice and ambulatory medicine, Bright Futures Periodicity Schedule Workgroup. 2017 recommendations for preventive pediatric health care. Pediatrics 2017. http://dx.doi.org/10.1542/peds.2015-3908.

100. Ramos-Gomez FJ. A model for community-based pediatric oral heath: Implementation of an Infant Oral Care Program. Int J Dent 2014;2014:9.

101. Albino J, Tiwari T. Preventing childhood caries: a review of recent behavioral research. J Dent Res 2016;95(1):35–42.

102. Borrelli B, Tooley EM, Scott-Sheldon LAJ. Motivational interviewing for parent-child health interventions: a systematic review and meta-analysis. Pediatr Dent 2015;37(3):254–65.

103. Merrick J, Chong A, Parker E, et al. Reducing disease burden and health inequalities arising from chronic disease among Indigenous children: an early childhood caries intervention. BMC Public Health 2012;12(1):1–6.

104. Centers for Disease Control and Prevention. About PRAMS, the Pregnancy Risk Assessment Monitoring System. Available at: http://www.cdc.gov/prams/aboutprams.htm. Accessed September 30, 2016.

105. Shearer DM, Thomson WM. Intergenerational continuity in oral health: a review. Community Dent Oral Epidemiol 2010;38(6):479–86.

106. Casamassimo PS, Lee JY, Marazita ML, et al. Improving children's oral health: an interdisciplinary research framework. J Dent Res 2014;93(10):938–42.

107. Center to Address Disparities in Oral Health. Centering Pregnancy Oral Health Promotion Extension (CPOPE) study. Available at: http://www.cando.ucsf.edu/cpope. Accessed December 20, 2016.

Social Determinants of Pediatric Oral Health

Marcio A. da Fonseca, DDS, MS*, David Avenetti, DDS, MSD, MPH

KEYWORDS

- Public health • Social determinants • Oral health • Children • Pediatrics
- Inequalities • Health promotion • Risk factors

KEY POINTS

- There are significant oral health inequalities among children and a biologic approach to oral health intervention neglects the role of the social environment on oral health outcomes.
- Oral health is significantly affected by social determinants and the conditions in which people live, which include socioeconomic status (SES), family structure, social environment, and culture, among others.
- Interventions to improve oral health must address the interaction between multiple levels of risk factors in the socioecological and life course frameworks.

Functional health trajectories in adulthood are shaped by childhood health and socioeconomic circumstances; unhealthy and socioeconomically disadvantaged children are more likely to become unhealthy, disadvantaged adults.[1] Chronic diseases are now studied within a life course framework that considers health issues a consequence of exposure to damaging experiences in critical periods of life or accumulated over time.[1,2] Therefore, starting in utero, important developmental processes may be affected during critical periods, causing short-term and long-term effects, including on oral health. For instance, good chewing ability at 50 years of age has been related to regular dental care in childhood.[2] Furthermore, childhood patterns of dental visit influence later dental care patterns, providing a cumulative impact on oral health throughout the life cycle.[2]

The World Health Organization defines social determinants of health as "the conditions in which people are born, grow, work, live, and age, and the wider set of forces and systems shaping the conditions of daily life. These forces and systems include economic policies and systems, development agendas, social norms, social policies

---

Disclosure: The authors have nothing to disclose.
Department of Pediatric Dentistry, College of Dentistry, University of Illinois at Chicago, 801 South Paulina Street, 254 DENT, Chicago, IL 60612-7211, USA
* Corresponding author.
E-mail address: marcio@uic.edu

Dent Clin N Am 61 (2017) 519–532
http://dx.doi.org/10.1016/j.cden.2017.02.002
0011-8532/17/© 2017 Elsevier Inc. All rights reserved.

dental.theclinics.com

and political systems."[3] The socioecological framework proposed by Fisher-Owens and colleagues[4] considers the complex interaction between personal and environmental factors that influence children's oral health, including individual biology, relationship within and between families, community and social networks/support, and the physical environment. It is also important to recognize the role these elements play within broader structures, including the health care delivery system.

Focusing on changing the behaviors of high-risk individuals (mostly on substrate, microbiome, and diet), which is the usual approach in preventive dentistry, has not reduced oral health inequalities; in fact, it may have increased them.[5] Most behavioral approaches to date have been weak because they tend to be poorly designed and atheoretic and have largely ignored social determinants of health; thus, the recommendations are mostly anecdotal.

Using caries risk assessment tools alone is not definitive because of their lack of precision, and the conditions that create dental disease have not changed.[5] It is well known that the best predictor for future caries is past caries.[5,6] Therefore, a different approach to establishment and maintenance of oral health in children, which leads to good oral health in adulthood, must take into account the many social and biological factors that contribute to the development of the disease. There is currently a limited body of evidence that describes social determinants of pediatric oral health. The existing evidence-base is primarily derived from medical research or research from adult populations, and recommendations for children are primarily empirical in nature. The purpose of this article is to provide a brief description of these social determinants and discuss areas for future research.

KEY AREAS OF SOCIAL DETERMINANTS OF PEDIATRIC ORAL HEALTH
Socioeconomic Status

Socioeconomic circumstances early in life help determine future health outcomes, such as presence of chronic diseases. In the United States, approximately 7 million children live in deep poverty and more than 1 million in extreme poverty,[7] which is known to stunt a child's growth and development. Low SES and neighborhood poverty are significantly associated with a greater risk of caries, unmet dental care needs, and poor oral health–related quality of life (OHRQOL) due to, among other factors, the following[8–12]:

- Low parental educational level and oral health literacy
- Less access to home and professional preventive measures
- Material deprivation (inability to purchase dental products, lack of running water, and so forth)
- Poor dietary and oral hygiene habits
- Less social support
- Employment issues

Consequently, children of low-income families are the least likely to adhere to preventive recommendations and more likely to have untreated dental caries and poorer oral health than their high-SES counterparts.[6,13,14] Children from high-income and high-education families have a better OHRQOL,[15] whereas those whose mothers are wealthier and more educated have a higher rate of dental visits.[16] Listl and colleagues[2] showed that the number of books in the household, used as an SES proxy measure, had a significant influence on good oral health in midadulthood to late adulthood. Furthermore, children of migrant parents, who tend to come from a disadvantaged background, also have a poorer OHRQOL and face significant barriers to access dental services, mainly lack of financial resources, to pay for treatment.[17] Not all studies agree, however, Carvalho and colleagues[18] did not find a significant association between caries development and household monthly income in Brazil.

Early socioeconomic inequalities have a long-lasting effect on systemic and oral health, with several important oral health indicators persisting into the third decade of life.[6] Peres and colleagues[19] showed that experiencing poverty in childhood led to compromised oral health in adolescents, even if there was an upward change in SES later. Adolescents who were always poor had the most caries experience and presented a low frequency of tooth brushing, leading to low exposure to fluoride and less effective dental cleanings. Adults who experienced a downward SES trajectory also presented poorer oral hygiene, more missing teeth, and high levels of untreated caries.[6] Most importantly, once disadvantaged children who had good oral care throughout early life ages out of the public aid system in certain countries, such as the United States, it is unlikely they maintain good oral health due to the inability to afford private dental coverage.[6]

Mothers who have good prenatal care tend to take their children to the dentist regularly and instill routine tooth brushing habits.[16] Unfortunately, poverty can affect pregnancy outcomes through inadequate prenatal care, maternal malnourishment, high maternal cortisol levels due to stress, and so forth. Therefore, these factors may have a negative affect on the development of the dentition and the craniofacial complex. Masterson and Sabbah[20] showed that biological markers of maternal exposure to chronic stress (ie, allostatic load) were linked to childhood caries experience and negatively associated with breastfeeding and other caretaking behaviors, such as taking a child to a dentist. Thus, the cumulative effect of stress over the life course may affect a mother's ability to provide optimal caring behaviors related to HER children's caries experience. Boyce and colleagues,[21] examining stress-related psychobiological processes that may lead to higher caries experience in low-SES children, found that elevated salivary cortisol levels, which are associated with stress, lead to thinner, softer dental enamel.

Malnourishment affects dental development, causing enamel hypoplasia, which increases adherence of cariogenic bacteria to the enamel surfaces, facilitating caries development. Some investigators[22–24] found a strong correlation between very low birth weight and enamel defects. Adolescents born with very low weight were at higher risk for enamel defects in the permanent incisors and first molars because their formation begins at birth.[25] Many researchers, however, failed to find a significant association between low birth weight, preterm birth, or small for gestational age and the prevalence of dental caries in young children.[26–28] Premature Japanese children had a 40% decrease in the prevalence of dental caries, which may have been due to delayed tooth eruption and good medical care in a developed country.[26] Saraiva and colleagues[28] found a significant positive association between preterm birth and dental caries in Brazil. Other investigators found that prematurity was not associated with dental emergence patterns but rather with biological (birth height and stunting) and nutritional (postnatal malnourishment) factors.[29]

Malnourished children tend to have more dental caries in both dentitions than their healthy peers.[30–33] Protein energy malnutrition, which is a deficiency in protein, energy foods, or both, relative to the body's needs,[34] can compromise a child's ability to immunologically fight dental caries.[35] In Brazil, underweight children were approximately 6 times more likely to have caries than children of normal height and weight.[36] Vitamin D is important for the proper formation of enamel and dentin and for the production of antimicrobial peptides, such as defensins and cathelicidin.[37] Therefore, its deficiency during pregnancy and early years may also lead to dental developmental issues. Children with caries had mothers with significantly lower levels of vitamin D than those children who were caries-free.[38] Another study showed that women who took high levels of vitamin D supplementation during pregnancy were more likely to report no caries in their children than women who did not take supplementation.[39] In contrast, some investigators[40] found no evidence of an association between vitamin D status and dental caries in children.

The lack of ability to purchase healthy foods is an important consideration in pediatric oral health because the presence of cariogenic substrate is one of the key components in the development of dental caries. The most commonly consumed foods by disadvantaged African American children in Detroit were (1) cold cereal, (2) potato chips, (3) sliced cheese, (4) bread/toast, (5) bologna, and (6) ketchup,[41] with soda consumption a significant predictor of dental caries progression in their primary teeth.[42] There are many potential explanations for this nutritional pattern. Low-income, rural, and minority families have limited access to supermarkets (food deserts), where there is a great choice of affordable foods, and hence make use of convenience stores that sell high-caloric and few fresh products. Lack of transportation to travel to a supermarket and neighborhood safety also add to the burden of acquiring healthy foods. High-caloric foods are attractive for poor families because they are cheaper, have a longer shelf-life than vegetables and fruits, take a long time to be digested, and require little to no cooking skills to be prepared, which these parents usually do not have. Furthermore, lack of appropriate cooking utensils and devices (pans, pots, stove, and microwave oven), utilities (gas, electricity, and running fluoridated water), and storage (refrigerator, freezer, and pantry) add to the problem. Chi and colleagues[43] reported that children who suffered low or very low food security had higher caries experience than those who lived in food-secure families, a problem that seems to continue into adulthood. A Canadian study showed that food-insecure working poor adults had poorer oral health compared with those who were food secure.[44] The former had a higher prevalence of denture wearing, toothache, pain, and functional impacts. On-demand bottle feeding at night and intake of sweet juices and snacks 2 to 4 times daily at daycare were also significantly associated with caries development in underprivileged children.[18]

Family Function and Structure

Family structure and stability are paramount for children to develop well and for the establishment of healthy oral habits. A family that experiences instability (eg, loss of resources, frequent moves, violence, child support issues, divorce, incarceration, or maternal depression) tends to have poor health behaviors. Maternal depression and stress interfere with the development of a consistent and nurturing environment due to loss of emotional and physical energy, less available time, less consistent parenting, less modeling of healthy behaviors, and so forth that likely affect the establishment of good oral hygiene and dietary habits and regular dental visits. Unstable families also have fewer financial resources and more competing demands, which may lead to less attention devoted to oral health. Dissolution of a couple's relationship can cause negative outcomes due to loss of family income and a great emotional impact on the children. If there is a high degree of conflict in the relationship, however, union dissolution may lead to well-being improvement for mother and child.[45] Furthermore, if a mother's sense of well-being and social support are good, the effect of the instability on the child's health may be buffered.[45] Children in single-parent households are more likely to have advanced levels of caries and have more periodic use of dental services[46] because the resources and social support must be distributed among all family members.[47] Family structure and household crowding also have a significant impact on children's OHRQOL, with single (only) children showing a lower impact of oral health on their quality of life.[12,15] Other investigators,[48,49] however, disagreed that parent structure was significantly related to oral health status.

In most families, it is understandable a child's health may be similar to the mother's because she has a central role in their development. Children may receive direct exposure to cariogenic bacteria through their contact with the mother so it is not surprising that there is a high caries prevalence among both caregivers and children.[11,42] Moimaz and colleagues[12] reported maternal education, family income, and frequency of dental visits as strong social determinants of caries in children and mothers' need for dental treatment. Goettems and colleagues[50] found that children whose mothers did not have regular use of dental services presented worse OHRQOL. In agreement with that was Camargo and colleagues,[16] who found that mothers who regularly scheduled dental visits for themselves and helped their children with tooth brushing also took their children regularly to the dentist. Low maternal education, which may lead to negative practices, such as on-demand bottle feeding at night, lack of assisting a child with tooth brushing, and dental visits for emergency situations only, increases the likelihood of an underprivileged child developing caries.[18] Corroborating this finding, Goettems and colleagues[50] showed that children of mothers with low educational attainment were more likely to have a delayed initial dental appointment and less likely to receive care after an initial encounter with a dentist. Therefore, maternal level of education may be more influential on good oral health than household income level.[18]

The influence of caretakers in the establishment of good oral and dietary habits in children is also related to mental health issues. Adults who report high depressive symptoms are more likely to have children who do not visit the dentist regularly,[10] and children of mothers who have dental anxiety presented more untreated caries.[15,51] Furthermore, familial use of deleterious substances also affects children's OHRQOL.[15]

Health Behaviors

One of the most researched social determinants of health is the role of culture and its influence on community, family, and individual behaviors. Culture relies on the embedded beliefs about the relative importance of health-promoting behaviors and the perceived risk of oral disease. Cultural patterns may facilitate the adoption of healthy attitudes, such as use of fluoridated water, positive breastfeeding practices, and a diet low in refined sugars, but they may also act as a barrier to adoption of these behaviors, such as resistance to vaccinations, resistance to water fluoridation, lack of understanding of the importance of primary teeth, and so forth. Dental fatalism of caregivers has been shown to be an important predictor of dental caries progression in primary teeth of low-income African American children.[42] As previously described, parental oral habits have a significant influence on their children's oral health. Many caretakers believe that good oral health means absence of oral pain; thus, they are unaware of their child's dental problems until they start interfering with the ability to perform daily functions, such as eating, chewing, sleeping, attending school, and so forth.

A child's sex may also influence oral health. Antunes and colleagues[52] reported that girls had a higher prevalence of caries and restorations in permanent teeth than boys, supporting the hypothesis that early eruption of teeth in girls leads to higher caries experience. A difference between gender roles and educational patterns, with a higher parental commitment to the oral health of girls, was also observed. Boys with high caries risk, however, eventually achieved the same pattern of caries distribution as girls. Two other Brazilian studies agreed that girls tend to have fewer carious teeth, better oral hygiene habits, and higher use of dental services than boys.[19,51] Lukacs[53] acknowledged the complexity of understanding sex differences in dental caries experience, with both biological (hormones, reproductive history, and so forth) and anthropological (culture-based behavior) playing a role.

Social Environment/Social Capital

The definition, measurement, and application of social capital have not been clearly defined, which has led to criticism of the concept and created methodological shortcomings in research.[54] There are many definitions of social capital, which has 2 distinct theories in public health: social cohesion (communitarian approach) and social networks (individual approach).[54] Social capital can refer to "features of social organization, such as trust, norms and networks that can improve the efficacy of society by facilitating coordinated actions."[55] The links between social capital and oral health can occur through diverse pathways: behavioral pathway (social norms, peer pressure, and diffusion of health-related knowledge), psychosocial pathway (stress-buffering effects through social support), access to dental care (community lobbying for access to high-quality services and promoting dental attendance), and development of public policies (political engagement and health advocacy).[48,54,56]

No systematic reviews on social capital and oral health are available, and there is limited and inconsistent evidence of the association between individual-level measures of social capital and oral health in children and adolescents.[54] Societies that are more egalitarian, independent of SES, tend to have better health because of their cohesiveness and support of individuals.[9] Decreased neighborhood safety and social capital, which are often observed in minority and poor communities, may restrict dental visits or reduce the establishment of dental practices, which tend to be located in safer and wealthier neighborhoods.[57] Several studies agree on the importance of social capital for the development of good oral health. It has been shown that individuals who live in neighborhoods with a high number of community centers report less negative children's OHRQOL.[9] Mothers with a low social capital index report more unmet dental needs for their children, showing less use of dental services and more dental caries progression.[42,56] Important predictors of caries development and progression in primary teeth of low-income African American children and their caregivers included social and community factors, such as neighborhood poverty and caregivers' dental fatalism.[42] Furuta and colleagues[58] reported significant associations between family social capital and oral hygiene behavior and between tooth brushing frequency and self-rated oral health in young Japanese adults. They also showed that higher levels of neighborhood trust and vertical social capital in school were linked with better oral health. In Brazil, community social capital was associated with fewer dental trauma episodes in adolescents.[59] Bramlett and colleagues[49] also showed a positive association between neighborhood social capital and self-reported oral health in individuals younger than 18 years of age.

Negative oral health outcomes can also be associated with high levels of social capital. Adults in Los Angeles neighborhoods with high levels of social support were significantly less likely to use dental care, but the underlying mechanisms for this association are not well understood.[60] In addition to that, Brazilian studies did not find a relationship between social cohesion and dental trauma in children.[61–63] Furuta and colleagues[58] argued that the association of social capital and self-rated oral health in young university students was not uniform. They found that higher trust was linked to better oral health but higher informal control in the community was not. Reynolds and colleagues[48] reported that children's oral health status was significantly associated with neighborhood social capital but not with family social capital.

The social environment is also important in oral health. Multigenerational families living within the household may provide additional social support. Households that can support involvement in community-based organizations and extracurricular activities show a higher resilience to environmental stress and show more positive outcomes.[64] Theories suggest this is based on social support, social capital, and decreased levels of stress within these households.[64] The school social environment has also been shown to influence dental caries of children. Students who participated in after-hours sports activities at school had lower caries experience, possibly because health-related activities lead to psychological and physical well-being and high self-esteem.[65] The same study showed, however, that school violence and theft were positively associated with dental caries.

Culture/Ethnicity/Race

Culture and ethnicity can also influence a child's oral health. Flores and Lin,[66] reviewing trends in racial/ethnic disparities in pediatric oral health, showed that suboptimal dental conditions were present in half of Latinos, more than one-third of African Americans and almost one-third of American Indians and Alaska Natives compared with only 20% of white children. In a different study, Hispanic children also presented the worst oral health conditions and lowest preventive dental care utilization, followed by black children.[57] This finding was explained mostly by the low maternal education and high family poverty in these groups.

Minority groups also tend to lack a medical home, which is essential for continuity of care and referrals to specialists. American Indian and Alaskan Native populations, for example, have a high prevalence of early childhood caries but are underserved by dental professionals.[67] A study on uninsured Latino and African American children showed that half of the parents were unaware their children were eligible for government health insurance, which caused the families considerable financial burden.[68] These uninsured children had suboptimal health, with 61% having unmet dental needs. Parental lack of basic knowledge of eligibility rules and of the application process, language and immigration issues, income verification barriers, and family mobility are some of the reasons for parental lack of awareness. Inadequate customer service on the part of public insurance agents, who gave incorrect information to parents, led to loss of insurance for 1 in 7 minority children.[68]

Migrant children and their families face multiple barriers to oral health education and access to dental services, including

- Fear of disclosing their immigration status
- Societal discrimination
- Low oral health literacy
- Cultural beliefs regarding oral health
- Communication issues (inability to use professional interpreters)
- Lack of cultural competency of providers
- Cost of dental services
- Lack of understanding of the host country health insurance system

A study of migrants in Australia revealed that women were not used to seeking health information outside their family and community, which led to their first contact with a dental service being for emergency treatment.[17] Furuta and colleagues[58] argued that cultural context may influence the way in which informal social control works.

Access to Dental Care and Workforce Issues

Access to dental care in the United States involves 2 primary components: dental coverage and dental utilization. The Affordable Care Act deemed children's oral health an essential benefit, which increased the demand for pediatric dental services and dental coverage.[69] Disparities by race/ethnicity and income persist, however: poor children and Hispanic children are the 2 groups most likely to lack insurance.[70] Barriers to dental utilization include a mismatch between demand for service and the supply of dentists who are willing to accept government insurance plans. Many do not do so due to low reimbursement rates and increased time spent filing claims and recovering payments. Moreover, most practitioners tend to establish practice in urban areas, neglecting rural and disadvantaged places where the need is greatest. The situation is similar for pediatric dentists, despite the increase in the number of pediatric dental residency positions in the past years.[71]

The recommendation that children see a dentist by 1 year of age is instrumental to help prevent oral disease and dental trauma and increase parents' oral health literacy. Despite that most children are treated by general dentists, however, most do not feel comfortable seeing infants and young children due to behavior management issues. To complicate the matter, there is a lack of pediatric dentists in many locations. Additionally, it seems exposure of dental students to pediatric dental procedures is decreasing in dental schools; thus, many graduates do not feel prepared to offer services for infants and children.

RESEARCH DIRECTIONS TO IMPROVE PREVENTION AND CARE

Traditional approaches addressing the microflora, substrate, and host/teeth are not sufficient to reverse the development of or prevent the effects of dental caries.[72] New interventions must focus on the entire family because adults' oral health habits have a great influence on children. The social environment of families must also be considered because that is where the health behaviors are developed and sustained.[5,42] Understanding chronic maternal stress as a potential risk factor for early childhood caries is important and should be considered in prevention efforts.[20] A significant body of health services research has explored the role of income and health inequality on health outcomes.[73] Both total income and a reduction in income inequality are suggested as having positive health outcomes, including oral health.[74] Small increases in family incomes could have a significant effect on reducing caries among young children.[42] With increased incomes, poor families can get better access to preventive services through better insurance. Furthermore, SES and maternal education strongly affect family knowledge and enforcement of oral hygiene and dietary practices.[57]

Increasing oral health literacy in poor communities to raise social and neighborhood capital, coupled with opportunities to access to care and improvement of the social conditions, may produce sustained positive outcomes in oral health. Broad system issues that lead children to lose insurance must be evaluated and corrected. For example, decreasing language barriers, better customer service from insurance agencies, and decreasing the bureaucracy can certainly be targeted for change.[68] More research is also needed to understand the role of social capital in oral health.[54]

The isolationist approach to prevention of dental disease, that is, the oral cavity is separated from the rest of the body, needs to change to a common risk factor approach with other health care professions.[5] Efforts to reduce caries risk among children should also be aimed at reducing sucrose intake, increasing fluoride exposure (through water fluoridation, professional applications, and consistent use of fluoridated toothpaste), improving access to preventive dental care, and creating an environment that helps maintain good oral heath across populations.[5,11] Migrant families need to be fully integrated into their new society and be given support to navigate a new health system. Dental professionals also must develop more cultural competency to better engage patients from diverse backgrounds in prevention, treatment and understanding of oral diseases.

Providing preventive dental services, starting at birth through community programs, home visitation programs, and pediatrician visits as well as using alternative dental providers, are important to prevent dental diseases. There is also a need to diversify the health care workforce; to expand interprofessionalism efforts between dentists, physicians, and other members of the health workforce; to conduct more research on oral health disparities among minority children; and to implement innovative solutions to eliminate these disparities.[66] The adoption of the medical home and dental home models focuses on integrating care and creating an environment with an ongoing relationship between the patient, provider, and family. A recent statement on poverty and child health by the American Academy of Pediatrics called all pediatricians to screen children for poverty and to connect those who screen positively to their community resources that can help alleviate the problem.[75] Dental professionals should embrace the same mission; just asking the question makes the problem visible, reminding the professionals of the complexities these families face trying to follow the guidance they give them.[7] For example, counseling low-income families to eat low-energy foods frequently is probably not realistic due to their access issues and lack of financial resources to purchase them.

Dental and oral health organizations must do a better job of engaging their members in advocacy efforts to fight for more funds for social and oral health care programs as well as for better reimbursement for dental care for poor children. Dental schools must continue to increase the role of community-based rotations to expand the students' knowledge, confidence, and experiences working with populations of greatest need.[76] It is also important to determine the efficacy of community-based interventions, such as dental examinations and dental sealants programs. Although these programs expand the number of children receiving those benefits, they do not guarantee an ongoing relationship with a dental provider. Additionally, there is no requirement that families complete treatment prior to enrolling in school programs, only that they present a dental form to the school in the beginning of the academic year starts. Watt[5] discussed several guiding principles to develop oral health interventions as well as examples of local and national upstream actions to promote oral health.

Interventions to improve pediatric oral health outcomes must adopt the chronic disease management model and a common risk factor approach to intervention. Addressing risk factors individually fails to address the interactions and complex pathways between these risk factors and oral health outcomes. Additionally, although individual intervention remains crucial, upstream policy interventions at the macro level are necessary to effectively address health disparities and inequality.[77]

SUMMARY

Developing good oral health is a major challenge, especially for minority and poor children. A radical reorientation in prevention of oral diseases is necessary to achieve sustainable improvements and to decrease oral health inequalities.[5] An understanding of social determinants of oral health is important to guide health promotion efforts; hence, oral health professionals must shift their thought process from considering only a patient's biological issues to a broader perspective of his/her social environment over the life course.

REFERENCES

1. Haas S. Trajectories of functional health: the 'long arm' of childhood health and economic factors. Soc Sci Med 2008;66:849–61.
2. Listl S, Watt RG, Tsakos G. Early life conditions, adverse life events, and chewing ability at middle and later adulthood. Am J Public Health 2014;104:e55–61.
3. World Health Organization Commission on Social Determinants of Health. Closing the gap in a generation: health equity through action on the social determinants of health. Final report of the Commission on Social Determinants of Health. Geneva (Switzerland): World Health Organization; 2008.
4. Fisher-Owens SA, Gansky SA, Platt LJ, et al. Influence on children's oral health: a conceptual model. Pediatrics 2007;120:e511–20.
5. Watt RG. From victim blaming to upstream action: tackling the social determinants of oral health inequalities. Community Dent Oral Epidemiol 2007;35:1–11.
6. Thomson WM, Poulton R, Milne BJ, et al. Socioeconomic inequalities in oral health in childhood and adulthood in a birth cohort. Community Dent Oral Epidemiol 2004;32:345–53.
7. Klass P. Saving Tiny Tim – Pediatrics and childhood poverty in the United States. N Engl J Med 2016;374:2201–5.
8. Schwendicke F, Dorfer CE, Schlattmann P, et al. Socioeconomic inequality and caries: a systematic review and meta-analysis. J Dent Res 2015;94:10–8.
9. Guedes RS, Piovesan C, Antunes JLF, et al. Assessing individual and neighborhood social factors in child oral health-related quality of life: a multilevel analysis. Qual Life Res 2014;23:2521–30.
10. Kruger JS, Kodjebacheva GD, Kunkel L, et al. Caregiver financial distress, depressive symptoms and limited social capital as barriers to children's dental care in a mid-western county in the United States. Community Dent Health 2015;32:252–6.
11. Reisine S, Tellez M, Willem J, et al. Relationship between caregiver's and child's caries prevalence among disadvantaged African Americans. Community Dent Oral Epidemiol 2008;26:191–200.
12. Moimaz SA, Fadel CB, Lolli LF, et al. Social aspects of dental caries in the context of mother-child pairs. J Appl Oral Sci 2014;22:73–8.
13. Capurro DA, Iafolla T, Kingman A, et al. Trends in income-related inequality in untreated caries among children in the United States: findings from NHANES I, NHANES III, and NHANES 1999–2004. Community Dent Oral Epidemiol 2015; 43:500–10.
14. Manski RJ, Vargas CM, Brown E, et al. Dental procedures among children age birth to 20, United States, 1999 and 2009. J Public Health Dent 2015;75:10–6.
15. Kumar S, Kroon J, Laloo R. A systematic review of the impact of parental socioeconomic status and home environment characteristics on children's oral health related quality of life. Health Qual Life Outcomes 2014;12:41.
16. Camargo MB, Barros AJ, Frazao P, et al. Predictors of dental visits for routine check-ups and for the resolution of problems among preschool children. Rev Saude Publica 2012;46:87–97.
17. Riggs E, Gussy M, Gibbs L, et al. Hard to reach communities or hard to access services? Migrant mothers' experiences of dental services. Aust Dent J 2014;59: 201–7.

18. Carvalho JC, Silva EF, Vieira EO, et al. Oral health determinants and caries among non-privileged children. Caries Res 2014;48:515–23.
19. Peres MA, Peres KG, de Barros AJ, et al. The relationship between family socio-economic trajectories from childhood to adolescence and dental caries and associated oral behaviors. J Epidemiol Community Health 2007;61:141–5.
20. Masterson EE, Sabbah W. Maternal allostatic load, caretaking behaviors, and child dental caries experience: a cross-sectional evaluation of linked mother-child data from the Third National Health and Nutrition Examination Survey. Am J Public Health 2015;105:2306–11.
21. Boyce WT, Den Besten PK, Stamperdahl J, et al. Social inequalities in childhood dental caries: the convergent roles of stress, bacteria and disadvantage. Soc Sci Med 2010;71:1644–52.
22. Gravina DB, Cruvinel VR, Azevedo TD, et al. Enamel defects in the primary dentition of preterm and full-term children. J Clin Pediatr Dent 2013;37:391–5.
23. Rugg-Gunn AJ, Al-Mohammadi SM, Butler TJ. Malnutrition and development defects of enamel in 2- to 6-year-old Saudi boys. Caries Res 1998;32:181–92.
24. Oliveira AF, Chaves AM, Rosenblatt A. The influence of enamel defects on the development of early childhood caries in a population with low socioeconomic status: a longitudinal study. Caries Res 2006;40:296–302.
25. Nelson S, Albert JM, Lombardi G, et al. Dental caries and enamel defects in very low birth weight adolescents. Caries Res 2010;44:509–18.
26. Tanaka K, Miyake Y. Low birth weight, preterm birth or small-for-gestational-age are not associated with dental caries in young Japanese children. BMC Oral Health 2014;14:38.
27. Seow WK. Effect of preterm birth on oral growth and development. Austr Dent J 1997;42:85–91.
28. Saraiva MC, Bettiol H, Barbieri MA, et al. Are intrauterine growth restriction and preterm birth associated with dental caries? Community Dent Oral Epidemiol 2007;35:364–76.
29. Bastos JL, Peres MA, Peres KG, et al. Infant growth development and tooth emergence patterns: a longitudinal study from birth to 6 years of age. Arch Oral Biol 2007;52:598–606.
30. Delgado-Angulo EK, Hobdell MH, Bernabe E. Childhood stunting and caries increment in permanent teeth: a three and half year longitudinal study in Peru. Int J Paediatr Dent 2013;23:101–9.
31. Alvarez JO, Lewis CA, Saman C, et al. Chronic malnutrition, dental caries, and tooth exfoliation in Peruvian children aged 3 – 9 years. Am J Clin Nutr 1988;48:368–72.
32. Alvarez JO, Eguren JC, Caceda J, et al. The effect of nutritional status on the age distribution of dental caries in the primary teeth. J Dent Res 1990;69:1564–6.
33. Alvarez JO. Nutrition, tooth development and dental caries. Am J Clin Nutr 1995;61(2):410S–6S.
34. Agarwal PK, Agarwal KN, Agarwal DK. Biochemical changes in saliva of malnourished children. Am J Clin Nutr 1984;39:181–4.
35. Rodrigues Ribeiro T, Shangela da Silva Alves K, de Miranda Mota AC, et al. Caries experience, mutans streptococci and total protein concentrations in children with protein-energy undernutrition. Austr Dent J 2014;59:106–13.
36. Oliveira LB, Sheiham A, Bonecker M. Exploring the association of dental caries with social factors and nutritional status in Brazilian school children. Eur J Oral Sci 2008;116:37–43.

37. Grant WB. A review of the role of the solar Ultraviolet-B irradiance and vitamin D in reducing risk of dental caries. Dermatoendocrinol 2011;3:193–8.

38. Schroth RJ, Lavelle C, Tate R, et al. Prenatal vitamin D and dental caries in infants. Pediatrics 2014;133:e1277–84.

39. Tanaka K, Hitsumoto S, Miyake Y, et al. Higher vitamin D intake during pregnancy is associated with reduced risk of dental caries in young Japanese children. Ann Epidemiol 2015;25:620–5.

40. Herzog K, Scott JM, Hujoel P, et al. Association of vitamin D and dental caries in children: findings from the National Health and Nutrition Examination Survey, 2005-2006. J Am Dent Assoc 2016;147:413–20.

41. Kolker JL, Yuan Y, Burt BA, et al. Dental caries and dietary patterns in low-income African American children. Pediatr Dent 2007;29:457–64.

42. Ismail AI, Sohn W, Lim S, et al. Predictors of dental caries progression in primary teeth. J Dent Res 2009;88:270–5.

43. Chi DL, Masterson EE, Carle AC, et al. Socioeconomic status, food security, and dental caries in US children: mediation analyses of data from the National Health and Nutrition Examination Survey, 2007-2008. Am J Public Health 2014;104: 860–4.

44. Muirhead V, Quinonez C, Figueiredo R, et al. Oral health disparities and food insecurity in working poor Canadians. Community Dent Oral Epidemiol 2009; 37:294–304.

45. Bzostek SH, Beck AN. Familial instability and young children's physical health. Soc Sci Med 2011;73:282–92.

46. Mattila ML, Rautava P, Sillanpaa M, et al. Caries in five-year-old children and associations with family-related factors. J Dent Res 2000;79:875–81.

47. Aday LA, Forthofer RN. A profile of black and Hispanic subgroups' access to dental care: findings from the National Health Interview Survey. J Public Health Dent 1992;52:210–5.

48. Reynolds JC, Damiano PC, Glanville JL, et al. Neighborhood and family social capital and parent-reported oral health of children in Iowa. Community Dent Oral Epidemiol 2015;43:569–77.

49. Bramlett MD, Soobader MJ, Fisher-Owens SA, et al. Assessing a multilevel model of young children's oral health with national survey data. Community Dent Oral Epidemiol 2010;38:287–98.

50. Goettems ML, Ardenghi TM, Demarco FF, et al. Children's use of dental services: influence of maternal dental anxiety, attendance pattern, and perception of children's quality of life. Community Dent Oral Epidemiol 2012;40:451–8.

51. Goettems ML, Ardenghi TM, Romano AR, et al. Influence of maternal anxiety on the child's dental caries experience. Caries Res 2012;46:3–8.

52. Antunes JL, Junqueira SR, Frazao P, et al. City-level gender differentials in the prevalence of dental caries and restorative dental treatment. Health Place 2003;9:231–9.

53. Lukacs JR. Sex differences in dental caries experience: clinical evidence, complex etiology. Clin Oral Investig 2011;15:649–56.

54. Rouxel PL, Heilmann A, Aida J, et al. Social capital: theory, evidence, and implications for oral health. Community Dent Oral Epidemiol 2015;43:97–105.

55. Putnam RD. The prosperous community: social capital and public life. Am Prospect 1993;4:35–42.

56. Iida H, Rozier RG. Mother-perceived social capital and children's oral health and use of dental care in the United States. Am J Public Health 2013;103:480–7.

57. Guarnizo-Herreno CC, Wehby GL. Explaining racial/ethnic disparities in children's dental health: a decomposition analysis. Am J Public Health 2012;102: 859–66.

58. Furuta M, Ekuni D, Takao S, et al. Social capital and self-rated oral health among young people. Community Dent Oral Epidemiol 2012;40:97–104.

59. Patussi MP, Hardy R, Sheiham A. Neighborhood social capital and dental injuries in Brazilian adolescents. Am J Public Health 2006;96:1462–8.

60. Chi DL, Carpiano RM. Neighborhood social capital, neighborhood attachment, and dental care use for Los Angeles family and neighborhood survey adults. Am J Public Health 2013;103:e88–95.

61. Moyses SJ, Moyses ST, McCarthy M, et al. Intra-urban differentials in child dental trauma in relation to healthy cities policies in Curitiba, Brazil. Health Place 2006; 12:48–64.

62. De Paiva HN, Paiva PC, de Paula Silva CJ, et al. Is there an association between traumatic dental injury and social capital, binge drinking and socioeconomic indicators among schoolchildren? PLoS One 2015;10:e0118484.

63. Patussi MP, Marcenes W, Croucher R, et al. Social deprivation, income inequality, social cohesion, and dental caries in Brazilian school children. Soc Sci Med 2001; 53:915–25.

64. Attree P, French B, Milton B, et al. The experience of community engagement for individuals: a rapid review of evidence. Health Soc Care Community 2011;19: 250–60.

65. Fernandez MR, Goettems ML, Ardenghi TM, et al. The role of school social environment on dental caries experience in 8- to 12-year-old Brazilian children: a multilevel analysis. Caries Res 2015;49:548–56.

66. Flores G, Lin H. Trends in racial/ethnic disparities in medical and oral health, access to care, and use of services in US children: has anything changed over the years? Int J Equity Health 2013;12:10.

67. Braun PA, Lind KE, Batliner T, et al. Caregiver reported oral health-related quality of life in young American Indian children. J Immigr Minor Health 2014;16: 951–8.

68. Flores G, Lin H, Walker C, et al. A cross-sectional study of parental awareness of and reasons for lack of health insurance among minority children, and the impact on health, access to care, and unmet needs. Int J Equity Health 2016; 15:44.

69. Vujicic M, Yarbrough C, Nasseh K. The effect of the Affordable Care Act's expanded coverage policy on access to dental care. Med Care 2014;52:715–9.

70. Berdahl TA, Friedman BS, McCormick MC, et al. Annual report on health care for children and youth in the United States: trends in racial/ethnic, income, and insurance disparities over time, 2002-2009. Acad Pediatr 2013;13:191–203.

71. Davis MJ. Pediatric dentistry workforce issues: a task force white paper. American Academy of Pediatric Dentistry task force on work force issues. Pediatr Dent 1999;22:331–5.

72. Selwitz RH, Ismail AI, Pitts NB. Dental caries. Lancet 2007;369:51–9.

73. Kawachi I, Kennedy BP. Income inequality and health: pathways and mechanisms. Health Serv Res 1999;34:215–27.

74. Watt R, Sheiham A. Inequalities in oral health: a review of the evidence and recommendations for action. Br Dent J 1999;187:6–12.

75. American Academy of Pediatrics Council on Community Pediatrics. Poverty and child health in the United States. Pediatrics 2016;137(4):e2–160339.

76. Mouradian WE, Wehr E, Crall JJ. Disparities in children's oral health and access to dental care. JAMA 2000;284:2625–31.

77. Watt RG. Social determinants of oral health inequalities: implications for action. Community Dent Oral Epidemiol 2012;40:44–8.

Intergenerational and Social Interventions to Improve Children's Oral Health

Mary E. Northridge, PhD, MPH[a,b,]*, Eric W. Schrimshaw, PhD[c],
Ivette Estrada, MA, MPhil[d], Ariel P. Greenblatt, DMD, MPH[e],
Sara S. Metcalf, PhD[f], Carol Kunzel, PhD[b,d]

KEYWORDS

- Children's oral health • Oral health equity • Dental caries • Periodontal disease
- Intergenerational interventions • Parental interventions • Social interventions
- Community-based interventions

KEY POINTS

- Community context and the influence of the broader social determinants of health such as education, race/ethnicity, and income are important considerations in achieving oral health equity for children.
- Intergenerational influences, including caregivers' attributes, attitudes, and knowledge, may be viewed as intermediary mechanisms through which societal and community influences affect children's oral health.
- Promising social intervention approaches to improving children's oral health include improving access to fluoride in its various forms and reducing sugar consumption.
- Linking community-based dental services with settings where children live, learn, and play, such as day care centers and schools, is important for oral health promotion.
- Integrating oral health education with supervised tooth brushing with fluoridated toothpaste or professional oral care practices may prevent dental caries in children.

Disclosure Statement: The authors have nothing to disclose.
[a] Department of Epidemiology & Health Promotion, New York University College of Dentistry, 433 First Avenue, Room 726, New York, NY 10010, USA; [b] Department of Sociomedical Sciences, Columbia University Mailman School of Public Health, 722 West 168th Street, New York, NY 10032, USA; [c] Department of Sociomedical Sciences, Columbia University Mailman School of Public Health, 722 West 168th Street, Room 907, New York, NY 10032, USA; [d] Section of Population Oral Health, Columbia University College of Dental Medicine, 630 West 168th Street, P&S Box 20, New York, NY 10032, USA; [e] Department of Epidemiology & Health Promotion, New York University College of Dentistry, 433 First Avenue, Room 715B, New York, NY 10010, USA; [f] Department of Geography, The State University of New York at Buffalo, 115 Wilkeson Quad, Ellicott Complex, Buffalo, NY 14261-0055, USA
* Corresponding author. Department of Epidemiology & Health Promotion, New York University College of Dentistry, 433 First Avenue, Room 726, New York, NY 10010.
E-mail address: men6@nyu.edu

Dent Clin N Am 61 (2017) 533–548
http://dx.doi.org/10.1016/j.cden.2017.02.003
0011-8532/17/© 2017 Elsevier Inc. All rights reserved.

dental.theclinics.com

INTRODUCTION

Dental caries and gingival and periodontal diseases are the most common preventable chronic oral diseases of childhood.[1] Both dental caries and periodontal disease are progressive in nature and initiated early in the life course, yet both are also largely preventable.[2] If left untreated, however, oral health problems in children not only cause pain and suffering and lead to oral health problems in later life, they also influence growth, development, and cognitive function.[1,3] **Fig. 1** presents the estimated number of people affected by common diseases, with dental caries (tooth decay) affecting almost half (44%) and severe periodontitis (periodontal disease) affecting 11% of the world population in 2010.

Widespread fluoridation of community drinking water in the United States has been credited in part with the decline in dental caries achieved during the second half of the twentieth century.[4] Among the striking results of this community-level intervention is that tooth loss is no longer considered inevitable.[4] Despite documented improvements for the US population as a whole, however, dental caries and gingival and periodontal disease disproportionately affect underprivileged, disadvantaged, and socially marginalized communities, leading to oral health inequities.[5,6]

Therefore, treating children solely in clinical settings and focusing entirely on those at high risk for oral disease is an ineffective strategy to reach the large numbers of children at risk for oral disease worldwide.[6,7] Dental providers ought to be aware of interventions to prevent oral disease and promote oral health that begin with effective intergenerational and social interventions, which are the focus of this review.

CONCEPTUAL FRAMEWORKS

Three conceptual frameworks with origins in public health scholarship are key to understanding how intergenerational and social interventions may potentially improve children's health at the individual and population levels and promote health equity. Each of these frameworks is presented next in a stylized version with accompanying descriptions and their original sources.

First, the life course approach is the study of long-term effects on chronic disease risk of physical and social exposures during gestation, childhood, adolescence, young adulthood, and later adult life.[8] For instance, in disadvantaged populations and underserved communities, poor nutrition, lack of preventive oral health care, violence leading to face trauma, and excessive alcohol and tobacco use may affect teeth and their supporting structures, leading to dental caries (beginning in early childhood), periodontal disease (especially in adults), and eventually tooth loss (particularly in older adults).[9] **Fig. 2** presents a simplified version of the developing dentition over the life course, along with health behaviors at critical periods that foster healthy teeth.

Second, socio-ecological approaches recognize the multidimensional and multilevel influences on children's oral health. Adapting the concentric oval design from the report, *Shaping a Health Statistics Vision for the 21st Century* by the National Committee on Vital and Health Statistics,[10] Fisher-Owens and colleagues[11] identified domains of determinants of oral health at 3 levels of influence: the child level, the family level, and the community level. A stylized version of this socio-ecological model, which emphasizes that tooth decay (dental caries) is a multifactorial disease that develops over time, is presented as **Fig. 3**.

The third conceptual framework is derived in part from a health promotion model that considers dynamic social processes through which social and environmental inequalities—and associated health disparities—are produced, reproduced, and potentially transformed.[12] Patrick and colleagues[13] drew upon this model as well as the life

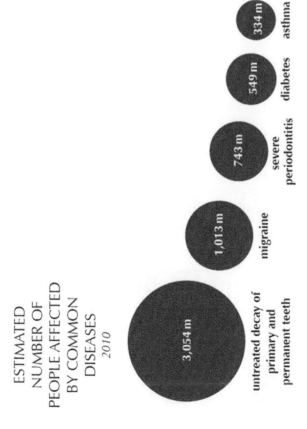

ESTIMATED NUMBER OF PEOPLE AFFECTED BY COMMON DISEASES
2010

Tooth decay is the most prevalent of conditions, affecting almost half (44%) of the world population in 2010, followed by tension-type headache (21%), migraine (15%), severe periodontitis (11%), diabetes (8%) and asthma (5%).

Fig. 1. The estimated number of people affected by common diseases worldwide, with dental caries (tooth decay) affecting 3,054 m people and periodontal disease (severe periodontitis) affecting 743 m people. (*From* The challenge of oral disease—a call for global action. The oral health atlas. 2nd edition. Geneva (Switzerland): FDI World Dental Federation; 2015; with permission.)

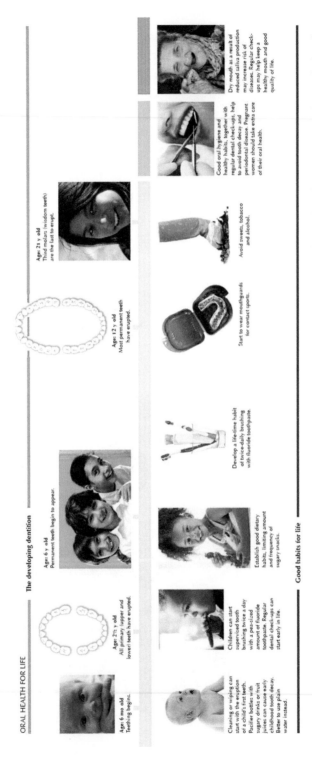

Fig. 2. A life course perspective on the developing dentition from infancy to later life, juxtaposed with health behaviors at critical periods that foster healthy teeth. (*From* The challenge of oral disease—a call for global action. The oral health atlas. 2nd edition. Geneva (Switzerland): FDI World Dental Federation; 2015; with permission.)

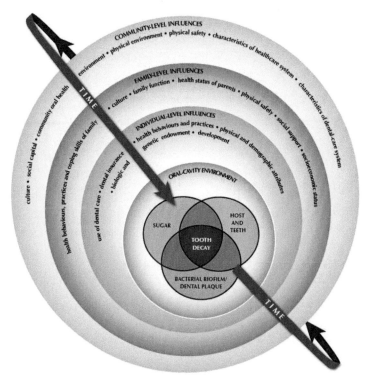

Fig. 3. A socio-ecological model of tooth decay (dental caries) as it develops over time, triggered by acid production resulting from the breakdown of sugar by bacteria, yet involving a wide range of other factors at the community, family, and individual levels. (*From* The challenge of oral disease—a call for global action. The oral health atlas. 2nd edition. Geneva (Switzerland): FDI World Dental Federation; 2015; with permission.)

course perspective to create an organizing framework for addressing oral health disparities. In **Fig. 4**, health and well-being at the individual and population scales (notably oral health and oral-related quality of life) are shown at the center of the graphic, and particular influences at the individual scale (health behaviors, type and use of services) and interpersonal scale (stressors, social integration and support) that relate to family or social factors are depicted in the next concentric circle, followed by community scale influences (social environment, physical environment) in the subsequent concentric circle, and finally societal scale influences in the square that contains the full model (macrosocial factors, inequalities).

INTERGENERATIONAL INFLUENCES

Broader ecological influences, including education, race/ethnicity, and income, and relationships with children's oral health outcomes such as early childhood caries (ECC) have received recent empirical attention.[14] Intergenerational influences, including caregivers' attributes, attitudes, and knowledge, may be viewed as intermediary mechanisms through which societal and community influences affect children's oral health.[14] For instance, an oral health study was conducted among a random sample of 457 mother and child pairs in Tehran, Iran. Findings were that twice-daily tooth brushing behavior and sound dentition in 9-year-old children were associated with

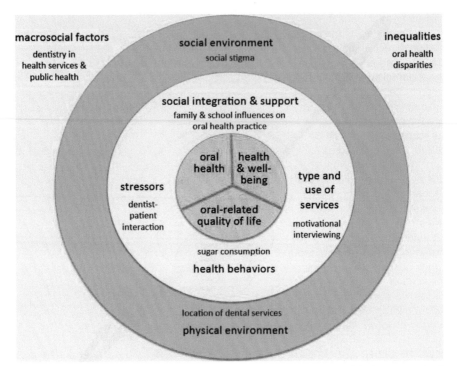

Fig. 4. A socio-ecological model of influences on oral health and health disparities, highlighting family and social factors. (*Data from* Schulz A, Northridge ME. Social determinants of health: implications for environmental health promotion. Health Educ Behav 2004;31(4):455–71; and Patrick DL, Lee RS, Nucci M, et al. Reducing oral health disparities: a focus on social and cultural determinants. BMC Oral Health 2006;6 Suppl 1:S4.)

their mothers' positive oral health-related attitudes.[15] Further analysis revealed that having sound dentition was most strongly explained by the mothers' active supervision of their children's toothbrushing.[16] Consequently, the authors argued that oral health professionals would do well to focus on the considerable potential of mothers in developing oral health promotion programs for children and adolescents.[15,16]

In a school-based randomized clinical trial of 423 low-income African American kindergarteners and their caregivers, results were that caregivers who completed high school were 1.78 times more likely to visit dentists compared with those who did not complete high school, which in turn was associated with 5.78 times greater odds of dental visits among their children.[17] These findings confirm the role of caregiver education in child dental caries and indicate that caregiver behavioral factors are important mediators of this relationship.[17]

In contrast, maternal stress and anxiety can negatively affect child caretaking behaviors and child oral health. In an analysis of data from the Third National Health and Nutrition Examination Survey (NHANES), findings were that children of mothers with an allostatic load (AL) index of at least 2, an indicator of chronic stress, were significantly more likely to have not been breastfed and to have dental caries than were children of mothers with a normal AL, before adjusting for socioeconomic status.[18]

A cross-sectional study with 608 mother–child dyads during the Children's National Immunization Campaign in Pelotas, Brazil, was performed.[19] Findings were that children from anxious mothers were more likely to present with untreated caries even after covariate adjustment.[19] Likewise, in a cross-sectional study among 187 mother–child pairs recruited from those seeking dental treatment in Udaipur, India, mothers of younger children and those with lower education and lower family income reported higher dental anxiety scores.[20] Moreover, a strong positive relationship was found between maternal dental anxiety and children's dental caries experience.[20]

In a systematic review of the literature on parental influence and the development of caries in children aged 0 to 6 years, the authors concluded that most research to date has focused on the association between caries and socio-demographic and feeding factors, with few studies exploring parents' attributes, attitudes, knowledge, and beliefs.[14] Nonetheless, there is research that suggests collaboration between psychologists and dental professionals may accelerate the identification and understanding of mechanisms that underlie risk associated with children's oral disease.[14] For instance, a cross-sectional study consisting of 92 parent–child dyads (46 cases with childhood caries and 46 controls who were caries-free) was conducted in The Hague, the Netherlands among 5 to 6 year old children of Dutch, Moroccan, and Turkish origin presenting at a pediatric dental center.[21] Findings were that parents' internal belief of their ability to control their children's dental health and observed positive parenting practices on the dimensions of positive involvement, encouragement, and problem-solving were important indicators of dental health in Dutch, Moroccan, and Turkish origin children, suggesting that interventions at the family level may reduce caries levels in children, especially those at high risk.[21]

VIEWS OF OLDER ADULTS

Older adults are important in advancing pediatric oral health, since they are both role models and caregivers of young children. As part of an ongoing study to understand factors at the individual, interpersonal, and community scales that serve as barriers and facilitators to oral health and health care among racial/ethnic minority older adults, 24 focus groups were conducted with 194 African American, Dominican, and Puerto Rican adults aged 50 years and older living in northern Manhattan, New York. Older adults were approached and screened for potential participation in senior centers and other places where older adults gather in the communities of Central Harlem, East Harlem, and Washington Heights. Just over half (54%) of the focus group participants were women, and just under half (49%) were predominantly Spanish speaking. Details of the recruitment and screening process are available elsewhere.[22]

Following standard focus group technique,[23] separate groups were conducted based on gender, race/ethnicity, and history of dental care. Groups consisted of an average of 8 participants (SD = 2.4) and lasted an average of 1.3 hours (SD = 13 minutes). All groups were audio-recorded, and the recordings were transcribed for analysis. Groups were conducted using a series of semi-structured questions about the factors that serve as barriers and facilitators to oral health and health care. Among the topics explored in each group was the role of children and families, including if they "talk with their families about going to the dentist" and "anything that families do that discourages or encourages" them to go to the dentist. Although the goal was to solicit information on how older adults may receive assistance from their families, thematic content analysis[24] of the transcribed focus groups revealed that

1. Older adults perceived generational differences between themselves and their children and grandchildren in the experiences with and the importance of oral health.

2. Older adults sought to encourage and assist their children and grandchildren in engaging in better oral health and health care practices more often than they received assistance from family members.

Quotes from the study participants detailing their views of generational changes and the attempts they made to influence the oral health of their children and grandchildren are presented in **Tables 1** and **2**, respectively.

These findings underscore the observation that good oral health is accepted as a social norm in the United States,[4] even in disadvantaged communities, and that clinicians may usefully leverage the care and devotion of older adults toward their children and grandchildren in promoting improved oral health and health care practices.

INTERGENERATIONAL INTERVENTIONS

Motivational interviewing (MI) is a patient-centered approach focusing on building intrinsic motivation for change.[25] MI was originally used in treating addictive behaviors and has since been successfully used to influence the caries prevention behaviors of mothers on behalf of their children.[26,27] One proposed mechanism of action is greater compliance with recommended fluoride varnish regimens in families who receive MI counseling as compared with families receiving traditional education.[27]

Recently, a health coaching approach has been developed based on: an interactive assessment; a nonjudgmental exploration of patients' knowledge, attitudes, and beliefs; a mapping of patient behaviors that may contribute to disease progression; gauging patient motivation; and tailoring health communication to encourage health-promoting behavior change.[28] Although there is not yet evidence on effectiveness, this may provide an approach to working with adolescents directly and family members who may in turn promote the oral health of their children. This is important since analysis of data from a prospective cohort study of 1037 children born at Queen Mary Hospital, Dunedin, New Zealand, found that the children of mothers with poor oral health had themselves (on average) poorer oral health almost 3 decades later.[29] Standard questions about maternal oral health ought to form part of dental professionals' preliminary assessments of children's future oral health risk.[29]

As part of the Baby Teeth Talk Study in a remote First Nations community in Manitoba, Canada, grandmothers who are considered local health knowledge keepers were recruited to participate in a total of 20 interviews and 4 focus groups.[30] Three key findings pertaining specifically to culturally based childrearing practices and infant oral health were identified and explored (feeding infants country foods from an early age, use of traditional medicine to address oral health issues, and the role of swaddling in the development of healthy deciduous teeth) as a means of restoring skills and pride and a mechanism for building family and community relationships as well as intergenerational support.[30] Clinicians ought to be open to discussing traditional and cultural approaches to childrearing with the caregivers of their patients.

SOCIAL INTERVENTIONS

The social determinants (social influences) of children's oral health are covered in Drs Marcio A. da Fonseca and David Avenetti's article "Social Determinants of Pediatric Oral Health," in this issue, so this topic will not be reviewed here. Instead, the focus of this section is social interventions on children's oral health. An important systematic review on community-based population-level interventions for promoting child oral health was recently published.[31] Overall, the authors found evidence of low certainty that community-based oral health promotion interventions that combine oral health

Table 1
Focus group findings related to generational differences in oral health

Sub-theme	Representative Quotes
Braces	*These kids wear braces now. In my day, you didn't wear braces.* *My son wore braces. Both my grandsons wear braces. I don't know if this is the new thing. I even see adults with them.*
Home remedies	*...Our grandparents, when you were sick, they would go to plants and make you teas...Then when you finally went to the dentist it was to justify that the tooth was no longer viable...If a tooth loosened up, they would use a string, tighten it around the tooth and pull...That's not the way it is today, they've been able to improve that but that way of thinking has stayed in...you are coming out of a place where they just took out a tooth when they could have just corrected the problem.* *I know that my grandfather, when I was young, I was at school and 1 day a tooth bothered me, and then my grandfather said: open your mouth. He put in a string and pulled out the tooth...There were people who grabbed pliers and if the tooth was loose, they would just pull it...*
Parental prioritization of oral health: then	*But people didn't worry about it because I did not go to the dentist my mother never made the effort, not, not even (to) brush my teeth or anything like that, no.* *...Our parents did not concern themselves with these things...the majority of us are different with our children and grandchildren. Kids now go get their teeth cleaned every 6 months. Before that was not the case. It was bad—there was no guides around that issue...In other words. Things were done only when they were necessary but it was not customary to go every year, every 6 months, to the dentist.*
Parental prioritization of oral health: now	*...I suppose that the new generation will not have the problems we have had. Because our generation, at for someone like me who has the teeth of an 80-year old. And from when I was a kid, I was never taken to a dentist. I went as an adult and it hurt. But not now, look for example, at my grandchildren. My daughter, since they were born here—for her the dentist is the most important...those kids are not afraid of checking their mouths or anything because they are used to go from when they are born, from the moment they come out, they start getting that stuff checked...our mothers were our dentists: they would pull out our teeth with a string...* *...I have a daughter who is 22. 23. And she pays a lot of attention to, "Mami, you should go to the dentist." "Mami, you have to," to her sister, who is younger. "We have to take her..." She pays a lot of attention to that...Because, to be honest, I don't say too much to her. To be honest...She talks more with me. She is always paying attention. Paying attention to everything that has to do with oral hygiene.*
Importance of oral health over time	*...We have children walking around at 16 years old that they got no teeth in their mouth, apparently something is wrong with this age generation...I think is diet...Everything they eat has preservative in it they don't eat natural, they don't eat fresh...A lot of things that we eat have so many different chemicals, you know and things like that...My mother and my father have perfect teeth. I was the one with the cavities...* *I have noticed that with the time that is, passing by, for me in the past people worried more about their teeth...There are so many more illnesses that people concentrate more on those and forget about their teeth, because that is, not so important...because of diabetes I lost some teeth. But when I was younger, I did not think too much about my own teeth. I only began to do this when I got sick, that I realized that I was losing my teeth, then I made an effort that I said, this will be my priority. Teeth, first.*

(continued on next page)

Table 1 *(continued)*	
Sub-theme	**Representative Quotes**
School-based dental care over time	*Now, I went to a school where we had a dental clinic...They don't have that anymore. They don't have a lot of stuff anymore that they had in schools.*
	We need more oral education...when most of us here were school-age, you knew about the dentist...You knew about the dentist...You know today? Number one: they don't have a dentist in school...That's non-existent. We had that...We had that...If not and you came from a decent family, a family that could afford it, you went to the dentist.

education with supervised tooth brushing or professional preventive oral care can reduce dental caries in children.[31] Although interventions that aim to promote access to fluoride in its various forms and reduce sugar consumption hold promise for preventing caries, additional studies are needed to determine their effectiveness in community settings.[31]

A systematic review of oral health interventions aimed at Alaska Native children aged 18 years and younger found that few were tested within Alaska Native communities.[32] Nonetheless, community-centered multilevel interventions to reduce sugar-sweetened beverage intake among Alaska Native children were deemed promising.[32] Another systematic review was conducted on the influence of family environment on children's oral health.[33] The authors concluded that since parents' dental habits influence their children's dental habits, special attention should be given to the entire family, not only to prevent oral disease, but to improve quality of life.[33]

In a study that compared changes in parent-reported pediatric oral health-related quality of life between children with ECC and children who were caries free, findings at baseline were that children with ECC were more likely to have fair or poor oral health and were rated as having more pain and trouble with physical, mental, and social functioning due to their teeth or mouth versus caries-free children.[34] At 6 and 12 months following dental treatment for ECC, however, there were significant positive impacts on parental ratings of their children's overall oral health and physical, mental, and social functioning.[34]

In a systematic review and meta-analysis of the prevalence, etiology, and types of dental trauma in children and adolescents, even as the prevalence of dental trauma was variable based on geographic area, the overall prevalence was 17.5%, with a higher prevalence in boys.[35] The major reason for dental trauma was falls, which occurred mainly at home and most commonly resulted in enamel fracture.[35] Policies that may prevent and reduce the severity of oral trauma include

- Enforce regulations to increase road safety through the mandatory use of seat belts, child seats, motorcycle and bicycle helmets, and reducing the prevalence of driving while under the influence of alcohol or other mind-altering drugs
- Implement appropriate strategies to reduce violence and bullying at school
- Enforce the mandatory use of helmets and mouthguards to improve safety for contact sports
- Strengthen the role of dentists in diagnosing trauma as a result of violence and child abuse
- Ensure appropriate emergency care for improved post-trauma response[36]

FUTURE POSSIBILITIES AND RESEARCH DIRECTIONS

Dental caries are among the most prevalent diseases of childhood and are principally caused by sugar consumption. Thus, reducing sugar consumption as part of a healthy diet promotes better oral health and may reduce diabetes, obesity, and other unhealthy conditions. Policies for sugar reduction include

- Enforce higher taxation on sugar-rich foods and sugar-sweetened beverages
- Ensure transparent food labeling for informed consumer choices
- Strongly regulate sugar in baby foods and sugar-sweetened beverages
- Limit marketing and availability of sugar-rich foods and sugar-sweetened beverages to children and adolescents
- Provide simplified nutrition guidelines, including sugar intake, to promote healthy eating and drinking.[36]

To further reduce dental caries in children, universal access to affordable and effective fluoride and universal access to primary oral health care are key strategies.[36] There is little evidence in the literature that oral health education alone is effective in preventing dental caries, although select studies have reported improvements in gum health, oral hygiene behaviors, and oral cleanliness.[31] On the other hand, oral health promotion interventions combined with supervised tooth brushing with fluoridated toothpaste were generally found to be effective in reducing childhood caries.[31]

Future possibilities include multicomponent and multisetting interventions that integrate oral health with general health promotion and care where children live, learn, and play, delivered by social service and health care teams. Dental providers need to recognize the multiple influences of broader determinants linked to clinical oral health outcomes (eg, oral health knowledge, behaviors and practices, and health care systems, including psychosocial environments).[31] In the future, there may be less reliance on dental professionals and researchers to deliver interventions and increased reliance on, for example, community health workers, to create cost-effective and sustainable solutions for promoting children's oral health.[37] Interventions informed by theory, such as the health-promoting school approach, community capacity building, and community engagement, in addition to the oral health promotion frameworks presented here, would reveal best practices.

Research is needed to overcome the limitations in the scientific literature to date on the effectiveness of intergenerational and social interventions to improve children's oral health. In particular, it would be important to

- Conduct more studies in lower–middle-income and low-income countries
- Conduct more studies in regions of the world that are currently underrepresented in the evidence base, such as Africa and South America
- Include assessment of long-term follow-up after intervention, including adverse effects and sustainability
- Include strategies to address diversity and disadvantage in the populations studied
- Engage community stakeholders in intervention development and implementation
- Target adolescents as an understudied group
- Collect and report economic and cost-effectiveness data, which is especially important to policy makers
- Strengthen the scientific approaches used, including implementation science[38] and systems science[39]

Table 2
Focus group findings related to influences on children/grandchildren around oral health

Subtheme	Representative Quotes
School-based influences	...Two of my grand kids are in charter schools....You take your child to the dentist...They will send you a letter home, you know, to tell you about taking the child to the dentist. When I was volunteering in the system....I would show them the children...I would show them my partial and I would say this is what happens if you don't go to the dentist...And, I worked 25 y in 2 schools. I think I have affected enough people for the next coming generation. All I did was take out my teeth...
General advice to take care of mouths	I tell my children: take care of your teeth, take care of your mouth... ...My children are in Puerto Rico...when I call them on the phone I tell them that...to take care of their mouths.
Offer brushing and flossing advice	I give advice to my grandchildren...that you should brush your teeth well...every day. I tell my grandson that he has to brush his teeth, take dental floss and how he brushes his mouth too. ...Children in the morning should brush their teeth to avoid having to go to the dentist all of the time...And at night, before going to bed, they should brush too. After a meal in the afternoon as well.
Encourage dental visits	I think it [fear] comes from childhood, because children don't like to go to the dentist, and it's a struggle. I talk to mine about making sure that they [children] go to the dentist so they'll maintain a healthy mouth....You know, so I just have one of my kids that will not go to the dentist and he's had a chipped tooth since he was a senior in high school and he will not go so that's on him but all the rest of them have beautiful sets of teeth and make sure that they maintain them. So it's only one of the bunch—that's OK.
Inspect mouths and breath	...I talk with them [grandchildren] because I am always paying attention that—I open their mouths and observe their teeth, their molars, everything. I always try to make them pick up their toothpaste and clean their mouths 2 or 3 times per day. And I do the most I can. You need to clean it as often as you eat. ...I always think about a grandson I have. Very often, 2 or 3 times a day, I ask him, "Did you go brush?" ... "Then go brush up if you haven't brushed your teeth." ...And I say, "Come here. Breathe out in front of me. That's OK," after he brushes because if not, go back and brush again....one of the things that keep the most bacteria is our tongue.

Children encourage parents and parents encourage children	Well, what she [daughter] does, though, is she goes—whenever she goes to a dentist…she'll say to me: "When was the last time you get into a dentist?" "Well, sometime. I haven't been there in a while, you know, but I'll be going soon." "Next week, or in a couple of days, she'll call me, "Daddy: did you go to the dentist?" You know. That's one thing she does which is towards my health…. I have a daughter that stays with me at home…And when we are going to bed, I go and brush my teeth. And then I see that she doesn't move and I say, "[name], go to the bathroom. Go wash your mouth."
Use own oral health as a lesson	…I've explained to them [grandchildren] what happens to me so you need to take care of your teeth. Brush in the morning, if you can't in the afternoon, before you go to bed…the experience that we have in our teeth in our mouth we don't want them to go through the same thing you know that we are going through…We want prevent the next generation coming up our siblings, our grandchildren from going through what we are presently going through so if we educate in all aspects of life, we need to educate the upcoming generation as far as health teeth, you know, everything. …I tell my grandkids you don't want to be like grandma. Keep, take care, brush your teeth, brush the tongue, the top of the mouth…. Why do you have to fight with your children that don't want to, they don't even brush their teeth? And they're big and you have to be there 'brush your teeth so you don't end up without teeth like me'… I got to tell my grandkids…They say. "Grandpa: I got more teeth than you do." "Cause I smile and he smiles, and he's got teeth that I don't. Like when he asks me why I have no teeth and then I explain it to him. I talk a lot with my granddaughter and with my other grandkids. What I say to them: look, I lose my teeth because I did not wash them, let's go to the dentist, you have to wash your mouth, brush your teeth, brush them after eating, before going to bed, you brush them to ensure that what happened to me doesn't happen to you and they go do that…they say: mama, mama, look that I just ate and I am going to wash my mouth. They are trained to do that.
Institute oral hygiene habits	It's all [oral health] based on habit. Starting with school, that's the first thing they tell you, mouthwash, brush your teeth 3 times per day. That's the main thing…When my kids were little, that was the first thing I would tell them about…that's a duty. I live with my 2 sons and the first thing my kids have to do—because I taught them from when they were little—with cleanliness has to do mainly with their mouths.

- Undertake analysis that expands the understanding of determinants, moderators, and pathways involved in promoting oral health in children
- Explore relationships between and across multiple levels of influence
- Apply scientific rigor and quality standards to the design, implementation, delivery, and reporting of future intervention studies[31]

Finally, it is imperative that effective interventions are described in such a way that they may be replicated or assessed for suitability for use in other contexts, as per the constructs of the Consolidated Framework for Implementation Research.[40] Without losing effective components of the interventions, available information must enable adaptations to be performed to suit community needs.[38,40]

ACKNOWLEDGMENTS

The authors were supported in the research, analysis, and writing of this paper by the National Institute of Dental and Craniofacial Research and the Office of Behavioral and Social Sciences Research of the US National Institutes of Health for the project titled, Integrating Social and Systems Science Approaches to Promote Oral Health Equity (grant R01-DE023072). The authors thank Bianca A. Dearing, DDS, MPhil, for early insights into the topic and interpretation of the focus group findings.

REFERENCES

1. Jürgensen N, Petersen PE. Promoting oral health of children through schools—results from a WHO global survey 2012. Community Dent Health 2013;30(4):204–18.
2. Satur JG, Gussy MG, Morgan MV, et al. Review of the evidence for oral heath promotion effectiveness. Health Educ J 2010;69(3):257–66.
3. Petersen PE. Sociobehavioral risk factors in dental caries—international perspectives. Community Dent Oral Epidemiol 2005;33(4):274–9.
4. Division of Oral Health, National Center for Chronic Disease Prevention and Health Promotion, Centers for Disease Control and Prevention. Achievements in public health, 1900-1999: fluoridation of drinking water to prevent dental caries. MMWR 1999;48:933–40.
5. Jin LJ, Armitage GC, Klinge B, et al. Global oral health inequalities: task group—periodontal disease. Adv Dent Res 2011;23:221–6.
6. Watt RG. From victim blaming to upstream action: tackling the social determinants of oral health inequalities. Community Dent Oral Epidemiol 2007;35:1–11.
7. Watt RG. Strategies and approaches in oral disease prevention and health promotion. Bull World Health Organ 2005;83:711–8.
8. Ben-Shlomo Y, Kuh D. A life course approach to chronic disease epidemiology: conceptual models, empirical challenges, and interdisciplinary perspectives. Int J Epidemiol 2002;31:285–93.
9. Northridge ME, Lamster IB. A life course approach to preventing and treating oral disease. Soz Praventivmed 2004;49(5):299–300.
10. National Committee on Vital and Health Statistics. Shaping a health statistics vision for the 21st century. Washington, DC: Department of Health and Human Services Data Council, Centers for Disease Control and Prevention, National Center for Health Statistics; 2002.
11. Fisher-Owens SA, Gansky SA, Platt LJ, et al. Influences on children's oral health: a conceptual model. Pediatrics 2007;120(3):e510–20.

12. Schulz A, Northridge ME. Social determinants of health: implications for environmental health promotion. Health Educ Behav 2004;31(4):455–71.

13. Patrick DL, Lee RS, Nucci M, et al. Reducing oral health disparities: a focus on social and cultural determinants. BMC Oral Health 2006;6(Suppl 1):S4.

14. Hooley M, Skouteris H, Boganin C, et al. Parental influence and the development of dental caries in children aged 0-6 years: a systematic review of the literature. J Dent 2012;40(11):873–85.

15. Saied-Moallemi Z, Virtanen JI, Ghofranipour F, et al. Influence of mothers' oral health knowledge and attitudes on their children's dental health. Eur Arch Paediatr Dent 2008;9(2):79–83.

16. Saied-Moallemi Z, Vehkalahti MM, Virtanen JI, et al. Mothers as facilitators of preadolescents' oral self-care and oral health. Oral Health Prev Dent 2008;6(4): 271–7.

17. Heima M, Lee W, Milgrom P, et al. Caregiver's education level and child's dental caries in African Americans: a path analytic study. Caries Res 2015;49(2):177–83.

18. Masterson EE, Sabbah W. Maternal allostatic load, caretaking behaviors, and child dental caries experience: a cross-sectional evaluation of linked mother-child data from the Third National Health and Nutrition Examination Survey. Am J Public Health 2015;105(11):2306–11.

19. Goettems ML, Ardenghi TM, Romano AR, et al. Influence of maternal dental anxiety on the child's dental caries experience. Caries Res 2012;46(1):3–8.

20. Khawja SG, Arora R, Shah AH, et al. Maternal dental anxiety and its effect on caries experience among children in Udaipur, India. J Clin Diagn Res 2015; 9(6):ZC42–5.

21. Duijster D, de Jong-Lenters M, de Ruiter C, et al. Parental and family-related influences on dental caries in children of Dutch, Moroccan and Turkish origin. Community Dent Oral Epidemiol 2015;43(2):152–62.

22. Northridge ME, Shedlin M, Schrimshaw EW, et al. Recruitment of racial/ethnic minority older adults through community sites for focus group discussions. BMC Public Health, in press

23. Krueger RA, Casey MA. Focus groups: a practical guide for applied research. 4th edition. Thousand Oaks (CA): Sage Publications; 2009.

24. Boyatzis RE. Transforming qualitative information: thematic analysis and code development. Thousand Oaks (CA): Sage Publications; 1998.

25. Borrelli B, Tooley EM, Scott-Sheldon LA. Motivational interviewing for parent-child health interventions: a systematic review and meta-analysis. Pediatr Dent 2015; 37(3):254–65.

26. Albino J, Tiwari T. Preventing childhood caries: a review of recent behavioral research. J Dent Res 2016;95(1):35–42.

27. Weinstein P, Harrison R, Benton T. Motivating mothers to prevent caries: confirming the beneficial effect of counseling. J Am Dent Assoc 2006;137(6):789–93.

28. Vernon LT, Howard AR. Advancing health promotion in dentistry: articulating an integrative approach to coaching oral health behavior change in the dental setting. Curr Oral Health Rep 2015;2(3):111–22.

29. Shearer DM, Thomson WM, Broadbent JM, et al. Maternal oral health predicts their children's caries experience in adulthood. J Dent Res 2011;90:672–7.

30. Cidro J, Zahayko L, Lawrence H, et al. Traditional and cultural approaches to childrearing: preventing early childhood caries in Norway House Cree Nation, Manitoba. Rural Remote Health 2014;14(4):2968.

31. de Silva AM, Hegde S, Akudo Nwagbara B, et al. Community-based population-level interventions for promoting child oral health. Cochrane Database Syst Rev 2016;9:CD009837.

32. Chi DL. Reducing Alaska Native paediatric oral health disparities: a systematic review of oral health interventions and a case study on multilevel strategies to reduce sugar-sweetened beverage intake. Int J Circumpolar Health 2013;72: 21066.

33. Castilho AR, Mialhe FL, Barbosa TS, et al. Influence of family environment on children's oral health: a systematic review. J Pediatr (Rio J) 2013;89(2):116–23.

34. Cunnion DT, Spiro A 3rd, Jones JA, et al. Pediatric oral health-related quality of life improvement after treatment of early childhood caries: a prospective multisite study. J Dent Child (Chic) 2010;77(1):4–11.

35. Azami-Aghdash S, Ebadifard Azar F, Pournaghi Azar F, et al. Prevalence, etiology, and types of dental trauma in children and adolescents: systematic review and meta-analysis. Med J Islam Repub Iran 2015;29(4):234.

36. Benzian H, Williams D, editors. The challenge of oral disease: a call for global action. Brighton (United Kingdom): Myriad Editions; 2015.

37. Northridge ME, Kavathe R, Zanowiak J, et al. Implementation and dissemination of the Sikh American Families Oral Health Promotion Program. Transl Behav Med 2017. [Epub ahead of print].

38. Lomas J. Diffusion, dissemination, and implementation: who should do what? Ann N Y Acad Sci 1993;703:226–35 [discussion: 235–37].

39. Mabry PL, Olster DH, Morgan GD, et al. Interdisciplinarity and systems science to improve population health: a view from the NIH office of behavioral and social sciences research. Am J Prev Med 2008;35(2S):S211–24.

40. Damschroder LJ, Aron DC, Keith RE, et al. Fostering implementation of health services research findings into practice: a consolidated framework for advancing implementation science. Implement Sci 2009;4:50.

Acculturation and Pediatric Minority Oral Health Interventions

Tamanna Tiwari, MPH, MDS, BDS[a],*, Judith Albino, PhD[b]

KEYWORDS

- Acculturation • Oral health behaviors • Immigrant communities • Access to care
- Cultural beliefs • Dental care utilization

KEY POINTS

- For immigrant children, acculturation can be a major factor having an impact on their oral health.
- Acculturation can be measured using standardized scales but more often is measured using a proxy, such as the length of stay and preference of English language.
- Improving the cultural competency of dental teams can reduce barriers to access to care for immigrant families and built trust in dental health care.
- Involving community members in oral health research design and implementation of research can be a crucial factor in the adoption of recommended oral health behaviors.

INTRODUCTION

Acculturation can be a critical factor in efforts to maintain the oral health of immigrant populations, in particular children. Although oral health disparities are often associated with these populations, acculturation remains poorly understood in the context of oral health. The purpose of this article is to evaluate the impact of acculturation on the oral health of ethnic minority children and the delivery of oral health care and oral health interventions to minority children.

"Acculturation as a term in anthropology comprehends those phenomena when groups of individuals having different cultures come into continuous first-hand contact

Disclosure Statement: The authors have no conflict of interest to disclose.
Funded by: National Institutes of Health, Grant number(s): 1K99DE024758; U54DE019259.
[a] Department of Applied Dentistry, School of Dental Medicine, University of Colorado Anschutz Medical Campus, 13065 East 17th Avenue, Room 104T, Aurora, CO 80045, USA; [b] Center for Native Oral Health Research, Colorado, Colorado School of Public Health University of Colorado Anschutz Medical Campus, Building 500, 3rd Floor, Suite 3000, Aurora, CO 80045, USA
* Corresponding author.
E-mail address: tamanna.tiwari@ucdenver.edu

Dent Clin N Am 61 (2017) 549–563
http://dx.doi.org/10.1016/j.cden.2017.02.006
0011-8532/17/© 2017 Elsevier Inc. All rights reserved.

dental.theclinics.com

with subsequent changes in the original culture patterns of either or both groups."[1] Acculturation reflects a shift in behaviors and lifestyle of people as they move from one culture and acclimate to another culture.[2] As a result of exposure to a new culture, some immigrant populations may experience rejection or, alternatively, may reaffirm their culture. In other cases, individuals may experience marginalization, which is alienation from both cultures.[1] The speed and extent of acculturation vary among individuals and have practical implications for health.

The effects of acculturation have been studied on systemic health since the late 1960s. Mixed effects have been seen on general health, health care utilization, and health-affecting behaviors.[3,4] In the earliest study to investigate the association of acculturation with oral health, the investigators reported that Mexican Americans with low acculturation levels had higher levels of untreated dental caries and periodontal disease than those with higher acculturation status.[5]

HOW IS ACCULTURATION MEASURED?

Acculturation is a multidimensional and multidirectional process and thus can be measured in several ways.[4,6,7] Scales commonly used by investigators include the 12-item Marin Short Acculturation Scale.[8] This scale focuses on the language skills, preferences, and ethnicity of friends in the participant's network. The Acculturation Rating Scale for Mexican Americans-II (ARSMA-II) measures the degree to which participants are culturally tied to Anglo and Hispanic communities.[9] This 13-item scale asks about individual preferences for thinking, reading, writing, speaking, and watching television in English or Spanish.

Acculturation can also be measured by a proxy variable, which most often has used questions related to English language usage by the individual. Other approaches have included questions related to individuals' preferred ethnic identity, place of birth, or residence pattern and sometimes may include questions on family values and gender roles.[6,7] Nativity status and length of stay are commonly used as proxies for acculturation measures and responses to these questions show high correlations with other standardized scales and language-based measures.[6] Proxy acculturation measures are most often used compared with standardized scales because proxies are easier to measure and less time consuming.

IMMIGRANT CHILDREN IN THE UNITED STATES

In the United States, 17.5 million children under age 18 were a part of an immigrant household in which at least 1 parent was an immigrant,[10] accounting for 25% of the 70 million children in the United States.[10,11] Hispanics and Latinos are the largest and fastest growing group of immigrants entering the United States. In 2014, approximately 55% of all first-generation and second-generation[1] immigrant children were of Hispanic origin.[12] According to the 2010 census data, Hispanic children accounted for most of the minority child population growth. The number of Hispanic children grew by 39% between 2000 and 2010.[11] Approximately 21% of US households speak a language other than English, and, within these households, 62% households speak Spanish.[10]

The other significant immigrant group in the United States is the Asian population. According to the 2014 Child Trends DataBank report, 17% of immigrant children are of Asian descent, and they are mostly first generation.[12] The top 5 countries of Asian immigration are India, China, the Philippines, Vietnam, and Korea.[10] According to the Pew Research Center, although Hispanic immigrants represented the largest community of immigrants living in the United States in 2015, Asian immigrants are growing at a faster pace and are predicted to become the largest immigrant group by 2055.[13]

This article discusses the effects of acculturation on oral health behaviors, oral health status, and dental health utilization for Hispanic and Latino children in greater detail than other immigrant populations. The focus is on Hispanic and Latino children because of the demographic significance of this group, which has implications for dental care delivery.[14]

HOW ACCULTURATION HAS AN IMPACT ON ORAL HEALTH OF IMMIGRANT CHILDREN

Living in a multicultural environment can affect both children's general health and their oral health when parental or familial attitudes, beliefs, and knowledge are different from those of the mainstream or general population. The influence of cultural beliefs is evident among immigrant communities and is strongly associated both with the length of stay and with the strength of social networks in the community.[15] Cultural processes allow individuals to become exposed to different ways of thinking about the world that may contribute to decision-making ability for their children.[15] As a function of intracultural variation, however, individuals vary in the manner and the speed with which they adopt attitudes, values, customs, beliefs, and behaviors of a new culture.[4] Children of ethnic minority and immigrant communities are exposed to a fluctuating environment with respect to cultural change. Such an environment of change may put them at a higher risk of developing dental caries because it may influence a family's and child's ability to cope with a potentially stressful situation, such as undergoing dental procedures and visiting a dental office.

The other common cultural component seen in ethnic minorities is a fatalistic attitude toward health.[16–18] It has been seen that ethnic minority parents who believe dental caries is unavoidable for their children may not actively seek preventive care and may not follow preventive recommendations because they think caries is an inevitable outcome for their children.[16]

Latino Children — Oral Health Knowledge and Behaviors

In Latino communities, acculturation frequently has been shown to predict oral health behaviors. The literature supports the concept that acculturation is a transition to a new lifestyle.[19] This transition can cause a shift in health behaviors, which may not always lead to healthier choices. In the case of oral health, acculturation may have an impact on the adoption of a more cariogenic diet, due to either lack of knowledge or easier access to processed and high-sugar foods and drinks. It is possible that immigrant populations may not even know the consequences of adopting these new diets. Horton and Barker[20] have demonstrated this scenario in their study of Mexican immigrant farmworker mothers. These mothers were attracted to infant formula provided by the Special Supplemental Nutrition Program for Women Infants and Child (WIC), which turned out to be cheaper than breastfeeding when they considered that it allowed them to work on the farms all day. Because the mothers were mostly first-generation bottled milk users, however, they were unprepared and lacked the knowledge of the oral health consequences of prolonged bottle feeding. They put sugary drinks in the bottle, gave the bottle to the child for prolonged periods during the day and sometimes during the night time, and were unable to wean the child off the bottle by year 1. Additionally, they were unaccustomed to the oral hygiene requirements of this new cariogenic diet. The amalgamation of all these behaviors led to high risk of dental caries in the children of these immigrant farmworker population.[20]

This pattern shows some similarities with urban-dwelling Mexican American mothers, although access to care is better in urban settings. A study looking at the oral health impact of maternal acculturation in a population of urban Latinas reported that strongly Anglo-oriented Mexican mothers were breastfeeding their children for longer periods, supervised their children during toothbrushing, and gave fluoridated water to their children. Also, Anglo-oriented Mexican American mothers enrolled their children in Medicaid. Exposure to sugar-sweetened drinks and higher consumption of candy, however, also were seen in children of Anglo-oriented mothers.[21] Similarly, Hoeft and colleagues[22] reported on urban Mexican American mothers' beliefs about caries. The study indicated Latina mothers had limited knowledge of dietary and oral hygiene practices. Although the mothers knew about some of the causes of dental caries, such as the use of bottle, juice consumption, and poor oral hygiene, they were uncertain about how these things were detrimental to their child's teeth and did not perform recommended oral hygiene routines.

Tiwari and colleagues[23] conducted a study to understand the oral health knowledge and behaviors of urban Latina mothers living in Denver, Colorado. Oral health knowledge and behaviors were similar to those reported in the Hoeft and colleagues[22] study; Latina mothers had limited knowledge about caries development and oral hygiene practices. In the focus group interviews, however, Latina mothers discussed cultural differences and variations related to oral hygiene practices and prevention visits. Most of them reported that children in Latino families might have multiple caregivers. Thus, maternal oral health knowledge and related preventive activities may not be practiced as consistently or efficaciously in Latino households. Also, mothers mentioned that they struggled to overcome peer and familial pressure when they took their children to a dentist for preventive visits. They said their family and friends suggested visiting a dentist if a child has pain and that preventive dental visits were unnecessary.

The behaviors and beliefs discussed previously, multiple caregivers in a family, and uncertainty of how sugary foods are harmful to children's teeth have a cumulative effect in deteriorating the oral health of Latino children. The authors speculate that exposure of the Latino population to a new culture and their partial acculturation —that is, alienation from their traditional culture and incomplete integration into the mainstream culture, may put them at greater risk for poor oral health–related behaviors.[19,24,25]

Latino Children — Oral Health Utilization

Acculturation also may have an impact on the ability of an individual to navigate the dental health care system.[2,6,26,27] Linguistic and cultural factors can play important roles in determining access to oral health services as well as personal oral hygiene practices. Cultural competency of health care professionals and the demands associated with living in a monolingual community may heighten the impact of acculturation on access to and utilization of care.[2] For example, Latinos who predominantly spoke English at home were more likely to use dental health services than those who spoke Spanish. Insufficient English skills may cause considerable difficulties and fears for Latino families, making them less willing and trusting toward dental care professionals.[18]

Valencia and colleagues[26] reviewed reports of Latino children's oral health utilization in Iowa. They found that less-acculturated Latino children were least likely to have a dental checkup in the past year and were less likely to be insured. The odds of having a dental checkup for less-acculturated Latino children were 75% lower and for more-acculturated Latino children were 40% lower than for white children. Also, the odds of having a dental home for less-acculturated Latino children and more-acculturated Latino children were 87% and 77% lower than white children, respectively. The odds of being insured for less-acculturated Latino children were 58% lower than for white children. Use of English versus Spanish was the differentiating factor between more-acculturated and less-acculturated families. Parents who responded to the questionnaire and interviews in English were considered more acculturated.

Another study reporting on dental utilization by children in Mexican American agricultural worker families in California produced similar results. Overall, the study participants had a high orientation to Mexican rather than Anglo culture; in other words, the caregivers were less acculturated. Acculturation was measured by ARSMA-II scale; 27% of the children had not visited a dentist in the past year, and 23% had never visited a dentist. Children who had visited a dentist in the past year had caregivers with higher US-oriented acculturation levels.[28]

Similar results were seen in a study of Latina mothers whose children were attending public schools and Head Start centers in 3 communities in Chicago. Acculturation was measured by Marin Short Acculturation Scale. It was seen that mothers who had a longer length of stay in the United States and had higher levels of acculturation took their children for the first dental visit at a younger age than did mothers who were less acculturated.[29]

Mejia and colleagues[30] reviewed the family level factors associated with lack of sealants in a California population of third-grade public school children. They found that 75% of Hispanic children did not have sealants. When the use of English language was used as an acculturation indicator, they found that children who spoke a language other than English at home did not have dental sealants as frequently as children who spoke English at home.

These studies have also provided some characteristics for the less-acculturated Latino families. They are mostly first-generation immigrants or recent immigrants, with shorter residency periods in the United States.[26,29,31] Parents of the less-acculturated children had lower education and income.[26,31] Moreover, lower levels of acculturation and length of residency in the United States seemed to act as a mediating factor in influencing a mother's beliefs about the importance of a child's first dental visit at a younger age.[10,29]

An interesting relationship of healthier oral health habits was seen in less acculturated Latino children, who were reported to have more adherent tooth brushing habits.[26] Another study demonstrated that immigrant Latinos enjoyed a considerable oral health-related quality of life advantage over the white non-Latino population.[32] This benefit was limited to first-generation or recent Latino immigrants.[33] Another study demonstrated that within a parent-child dyad, children who were US-born and more acculturated than their parents had a lower oral health-related quality of life than their parents.[33] As suggested by Sanders,[32] Mejia and colleagues,[14] and Acevedo-Garcia and Bates,[34] this paradox may reflect social protective factors operating within the Latino community. Latinos have high sociocentric values, and they value interdependence and readily internalize group norms. The transition associated with acculturation represents a move from interdependence toward greater individualism, which may erode the protective effect of these sociocentric values on oral health quality of life and healthy behaviors, such as toothbrushing habits and consumption of low cariogenic food.[20,32]

Despite some interesting findings to the contrary, less-acculturated Latino families experience multiple and additional disparities in oral health utilization than more-acculturated Latinos. These differences within the Latino population suggest that less-acculturated families comprise a particularly vulnerable subgroup that requires greater attention in increasing access to dental care.

Asian Children

There are not many studies in the literature that have studied cultural beliefs and levels of acculturation in Asian children and their families. A few that have dealt with these issues have revealed the influence of social networks in health care decision making and cultural beliefs related to traditional medicine.

Hilton and colleagues[35] examined the effects of cultural beliefs that could influence access to preventive oral health care for young children. They interviewed participants from several immigrant communities, including Chinese and Filipino communities. Lack of knowledge and beliefs that primary teeth are not important created barriers to early preventive care in all groups. Additionally, the concept of routine, preventive oral health visits was not widely understood, especially among older Chinese caregivers. Participants' fears of dental treatment also influenced attitudes regarding accessing preventive care for their children. The social networks of these communities also were found to play a significant role in health care decisions; grandparents, aunts, and uncles — as well as parents — were found involved in deciding when to take children to a dentist.

Wong and colleagues[36] examined the perceptions of Chinese parents regarding oral hygiene and dental care utilization. Parents' fear of dentists, lack of knowledge about best feeding practices, and cultural beliefs contributed to dental caries in their children and delay in seeking dental care. They were also highly influenced by their peers, who may oppose dental treatment or advice on seeking care in response to pain. Some parents also used herbal medicines and home remedies to treat children before they took them to a dentist. Similar beliefs were reported by Butani and colleagues[37] that Chinese communities tend to use a combination of traditional and Western medicine for oral diseases. Wong and colleagues[36] also mentioned that some Chinese parents might have trust issues with dentists and consider Western medicine more aggressive.

Vietnamese adolescents reported that oral health was important for social reasons; their appearance affected their confidence levels and ability to make friends. They were aware that sugar caused cavities and the associations between oral and general health. They valued dental treatment but still had some dental fear and anxiety.[38] Because the qualitative interviews in this study were conducted in English, the participants may have had higher acculturation. Therefore, a different set of approaches may be needed to educate parents versus the adolescent in these communities.

African Refugee Children

Children of other refugee groups that have been studied include those from a variety of African countries, although few of these have reported on the impact of acculturation on the oral health of these African immigrant children. One study reporting on dental caries status in African refugees demonstrated that African refugee children had only half the dental caries experience of either white or African American children. The investigators argued that these children had not been exposed to high amounts of refined sugars in their home countries. As these families undergo the process of acculturation, they may, unfortunately, adopt less healthy behaviors, such as consuming more foods high in refined sugar content. As a result, these children may be placed at higher risk of developing dental caries.[39]

Another study examined African immigrant parents' views on dental caries and dental health utilization of oral health care services. The study concluded that participants' cultural backgrounds influenced their decisions about their children's oral health. Respondents indicated that dental caries was viewed as a "harmless disease," because it is not life threatening, compared with malaria or HIV, for example, Consequently, it was not considered worthwhile to see a dental health professional. The more-acculturated parents in the study placed higher importance on the oral health of their children and were more motivated to use oral health services.[40]

Acculturation has some common effects on Latino, Asian, and African children that have emerged from the literature. Lower dental care utilization rates are seen in all 3 groups. The reasons for this can be varied; language can be a significant barrier in Latino and Asian communities, and parent perceptions and cultural beliefs can be common factor for all 3 groups (**Box 1**).

DELIVERING ORAL HEALTH CARE TO CHILDREN OF ETHNIC MINORITIES

From an ethnic minority patient's perspective, use of dental care services can be a complex process involving insurance coverage and affordability, accessibility of providers, provider availability, and acceptance of various types of insurance plans as well as provider interest in treating certain subpopulations.[41] Adding language and cultural barriers to this list further reduces the likelihood that members of ethnic minority and immigrant communities use dental care services. These factors can then lead to reduced trust in dental health care providers, which in turn may result in ethnic minority patients' not accessing care and not having dental homes.[41,42]

Language barriers heavily influence the patient-doctor interaction in dentistry. Use of interpreter services can improve provider-patient communication. Although dental researchers have reviewed the impact of language barriers on seeking/accessing dental treatment and preventive services, there is little research defining the benefits of interpreter services in dental care delivery.[43] Lessons learned from medical health care delivery suggest that interpreter services should be provided throughout care delivery and not just at the clinical encounters.[44] Furthermore, bilingual staff should be thoroughly assessed, and language proficiency assessments should be conducted before they provide services to any patients. Patient feedback should be collected periodically to access the quality of service provided by bilingual staff.[44] The medical literature also has shown that professional interpreter services have a positive impact on changing behaviors and improving uptake of preventive services by patients with limited English proficiency.[45]

Dental health care delivery is improved when dentists increase their awareness of patient values and beliefs because this awareness can have a positive impact on the effectiveness of doctor-patient communications related to preventive recommendations and treatment plans.[11,46] Overlooking the cultural and traditional beliefs of patients can lead to a lack of trust in treatment plan provided and further reduce the

---

Box 1
Impact of acculturation on oral health of immigrant children

- Higher acculturation, measured by longer stay in the United States or speaking English at home, increases the chances of using dental health services and can positively affect the oral health of children.

- Less-acculturated Latino families are an especially vulnerable group within the Latino community and may require greater attention.

- More research is needed, especially with Asian and African communities, to better understand their attitudes and beliefs related to oral health and utilization of dental services, including prevention services for their children.

chance of compliance by patients.[47] To be effective, delivery of dental care, including preventive dental services, should use a culturally sensitive approach.[47] Cultural competence is not limited to gaining information about the ethnic minority patients. Rather, it is defined "as an understanding of the importance of social and cultural influences on patients' health beliefs and behaviors, considering how these facts interact at multiple levels of health care delivery system."[47] It is important for a dental team to keep the cultural context of the child in view while providing recommendations to immigrant parents and to avoid stereotyped decisions. Cultural competency should be a critical component of dental education, and some dental schools have incorporated effective teaching approaches to address this goal. For example, using service-learning opportunities for dental students can help increase clinical interactions with ethnic minority patients.[48] Service learning also has been shown to improve cultural competency in dental students and may expose them to patients with different levels of acculturation within a culture. This early exposure of dental students to multiple cultures may help improve the understanding, knowledge, and respect for various immigrant populations and have an impact on their awareness of the role of the family and community in shaping the oral health of immigrant children.

The challenge of cultural competency is heightened by the lack of diversity in the dental workforce. According to the American Dental Association, there are approximately 196,000 dentists working in the United States.[49] Only 3.4% of the dentists are Hispanic/Latino, 3.4% are African American, and 7% are Asian/Pacific Islander.[49] The profiles for other members of dental teams are slightly more diverse: 6% of dental hygienists are Hispanic, and 4% are Asian/Pacific Islander, whereas approximately 23% of dental assistants are Hispanic.[50] Current efforts to improve diversity in the dental workforce include improving funding and scholarships for students from underrepresented groups and efforts to support recruitment and retention of ethnic minority dental faculty.[42,47] Attention should also be paid, however, to the cultural competency training of other members of dental teams, such as dental assistants, who are slightly more diverse. These team members are sometimes the first point of contact in dental care delivery and might be able both to create trust in the dental team and bridge language gaps.

ACCULTURATION AND ORAL HEALTH INTERVENTIONS FOR CHILDREN AND THEIR FAMILIES

Although providing linguistic or translation services is an excellent method of reducing language barriers, dental teams must go beyond this and pay attention to social and cultural determinants of health for immigrant families,[46] including developing culturally tailored oral health messages and oral health promotion to cater to the different levels of acculturation within the community. One critical component of oral health interventions for immigrant children is to involve the family, the community, and social networks in efforts to create better acceptance of interventions and to bring about sustainable change.

Cultural background can affect the motivation-orientation of individuals, their responses to health messages, and ultimately their adoption of new behaviors. Tailoring health messages in ways that integrate cultural norms and underlying psychosocial characteristics of the group can prove highly effective. Brick and colleagues[51] reported on the importance of framing oral health messages based on the exposure of the patient to mainstream culture. Their study demonstrated that immigrants who have greater exposure to the US culture, based on length of residency in the United States and whether 1 of the parents was US-born, were more responsive to gain-framed oral health messages. Participants who had a lower exposure to the US culture were more responsive to loss-framed oral health messages. Gain-framed messages communicate the advantages of engaging in a health behavior, whereas loss-framed messages talk about the costs of failing to engage in a health behavior. The investigators speculated that greater exposure to the US culture may drive more individualistic and approach-oriented ideologies and thus gain-framed messages are more appealing to these people. Individuals who were less exposed to the US culture may have more collectivistic and avoidance-orientation approaches and may respond more effectively to loss-framed oral health messages.[51] As discussed previously, many Latino cultures are associated with group norms and interdependence,[20,31] and less-acculturated individuals within the Latino community lean heavily toward these ideologies. Additionally, second-generation immigrants — that is, children born in the United States — may be more acculturated their first-generation immigrant parents. Therefore, it may be critical to think about oral health message framing when providing pediatric oral health interventions to less-acculturated versus more-acculturated communities. Oral health researchers may want to include questions, such as length of stay and if either of the parents was a first-generation or second-generation immigrant, to determine the level of acculturation of the parent before they design and deliver oral health messages.

Other methodologies that seem to work well with immigrant families are community-based participatory research (CBPR) and participation action research.[52] Interventions using these research methods enable immigrant populations to become partners in research. These methods allow the immigrant populations to shed more light on challenges and barriers faced by immigrant populations in accessing oral health care and to assist in the design and delivery of oral health prevention interventions that are culturally sensitive and thus more effective and sustainable.[52] Involving stakeholders from immigrant community in action research increases the cross-cultural understanding and thus provides an opportunity for both the investigator and community to work together to implement prevention intervention successfully. Recent oral health interventions have successfully used CBPR methodologies to involve stakeholders in research design and implementation of research and in recruiting and retaining study participants in longitudinal studies.[53–55]

Using community lay people who are trained to deliver oral health intervention, promote behavior change, and assist in navigating the dental health care system can help reduce the barrier for disparities population. These individuals are slowly becoming a part of dental teams and have various names, such as community health workers (CHWs), promotoras, and patient navigators. They have been used extensively to reach some groups, such as migrant farm workers and Latino and some Asian communities.[47,56,57] Several studies have successfully used CHWs or lay community members (who have been trained to deliver interventions) to engage immigrant parents in dialogue about accessing oral health prevention services, providing oral health counseling, and helping in initiating oral health behavior change through motivation interviewing.[54–59] A study that used a Vietnamese lay health counselor to provide oral health counseling to Vietnamese mothers of preschool children emphasized that similar cultural background of the counselor was an essential part of adoption of healthy oral health behaviors.[57]

In the Latino community, promotora-based pediatric interventions for oral health prevention are readily accepted and have been shown to ease recruitment of participants in oral health interventions, increase attendance for intervention activities, and retain the participants for a longer period of time.[55,56,59] Participating parents seem more comfortable in these setting and, therefore, may ask more questions than in a dental clinic setting, which in turn may help increase the understanding of oral health of their children and could also transform some cultural beliefs that do not support oral health. The success of these CHW-based interventions lies in that these individuals are familiar with the culture of the population in which they are working, speak the language, and are sensitive to the families' circumstances and thus are better able to meet the needs of that population.[53,54] CHWs can meet the parents/families outside of the dental clinic or even do home visits. This is a critical piece in engaging these families, because it reduces the travel cost for the patients and takes the conversation about oral disease prevention outside the dental clinic, where time constraints and other factors, such as language barriers, could limit this conversation.

Motivational interviewing (MI) that is successfully used in several oral health–related interventions is a methodology that holds promise for improving the oral health of immigrant children.[60] The first successful MI intervention to reduce dental caries in children was done in a South Asian Punjabi-speaking immigrant population in British Columbia, using lay community women to deliver the intervention.[58] Another recent study reported on the sustained effectiveness of a culturally sensitive, peer-led caries prevention intervention for Spanish-speaking Latino parents.[59] The intervention included components of MI, such as goal setting and participant-driven education. It also included, however, the elements of social and group support, which were appreciated by study participants.[59] It has been speculated that MI can help bridge the gap between the requirements of the Western dental culture and the cultural beliefs of the immigrant population.[58] MI's success may be attributed in part to that it is respectful to the cultural values of the participant and creates space to include spirituality and religious practices.[60]

Interprofessional collaborations between dentists, primary care providers, pediatricians, and public health programs, such as WIC, can be an innovative method to deliver oral health interventions to immigrant parents. These collaborations can assist in reducing barriers to accessing care; train ancillary staff, such as nursing staff and WIC nurses, to provide preventive oral health care; and conduct oral health promotion activities.[61] Immigrant parents use medical services at a higher rate than they use dental services. Providing some dental care, which may include oral screening for dental caries and preventive care at pediatricians' offices, can help immigrant families to access initial dental care, develop trust in a dental team, and hopefully develop a continuum of dental care.

The Vermont Tooth Tutor program was a good example of an interprofessional partnership to deliver preventive and restorative services to refugee children from Somalia and Southeastern Asian countries in Vermont. The program was designed by a collaborative team, including dental hygienists; community dentists; representatives from the Vermont Department of Health, local hospitals, and school of nursing; and a pediatrician from the school district. The implementation of the study was within the schools; preventive services were delivered to 60% of all the participating school children by the second year.[62]

Another program for colocation of dental and primary care providers has been implemented in Los Angeles County. This program is not aimed exclusively at immigrant children but is intended to overcome barriers to care for low-income populations. As a result of this colocation program, the participating Federally Qualified Health Centers reported increasing preventive visits by 3-fold; oral health education and fluoride varnish were provided during these visits. A significant increase was seen in treatment visits as well.[63] Such a model of care can be used to improve dental care utilization in immigrant populations (**Box 2**).

Box 2
Oral health interventions for immigrant families

- Understanding the motivation-orientation at the individual and community levels and designing oral health messages accordingly
- Developing interventions using CBPR methodologies
- Delivery of interventions using trained lay community members — similar cultural background of the health worker could be central in adopting new health behaviors
- Using respectful and nonconfrontational approaches, such as MI
- Interprofessional collaboration to bring all health care providers together to improve the overall health

---

SUMMARY

The population demographics of the United States are changing rapidly and at a pace that is faster than ever. With approximately 25% of children now belonging to immigrant households, it is imperative that dental teams update their cultural competency and that delivery of care uses culturally and linguistically sensitive approaches. A critical point in delivering dental health care and conducting prevention interventions with immigrant children is to include the families, the community, and their social networks so that interventions are readily accepted, and trust is established with a dentist.

Acculturation is rarely absolute but rather reflects a continuum. Exposure of immigrant families to a new culture can lead to different levels of adoption of the new culture; it may be influenced by the length of stay in the United States, language spoken at home, living in urban versus rural surroundings, income, education, and social networks. Acculturation can be measured either using a standardized scale or by proxy measures, such as length of residency and preference of language. The most common approach to measurement is the use of a proxy.

The extent of acculturation has an impact on oral health behaviors and oral health utilization. Higher acculturation increases the likelihoods of using dental health services and can positively affect the oral health of children. Children of less-acculturated parents may have poor oral health outcomes and lower health care utilization. More research is needed to understand the different levels of acculturation and why some families are more acculturated than others. For now, the authors speculate that income and education play a significant role in deciding how acculturated a family is, but other underlying reasons for these differences need to be understood as well.

This article describes several approaches that have been used to successfully deliver oral health interventions to immigrant communities. The oral health research community will be well served if awareness is increased of the cultural beliefs and backgrounds of these communities and if prevention interventions tailored to their needs are designed and delivered.

ACKNOWLEDGMENT

The authors are grateful for the ongoing support of their work by the National Institute of Dental and Craniofacial Research (U54DE019259 and 1K99DE024758).

REFERENCES

1. Redfield R, Linton R, Herskovits MJ. Memorandum for the study of acculturation. Am Anthropol 1936;38:149–52.

2. Stewart DC, Ortega AN, Dausey D, et al. Oral health and use of dental services among Hispanics. J Public Health Dent 2002;62:84–91.
3. Henry JP, Cassel JC. Psychosocial factors in essential hypertension. Recent epidemiologic and animal experimental evidence. Am J Epidemiol 1969;90:171–200.
4. Abraído-Lanza AF. Social support and psychological adjustment among Latinas with arthritis: a test of a theoretical model. Ann Behav Med 2004;27(3):162–71.
5. Ismail AI, Szpunar SM. Oral health status of Mexican-Americans with low and high acculturation status: Findings from southwest HHANES, 1982–84. J Public Health Dent 1990;50:24–31.
6. Abraido-Lanza AF, Chao MT, Flórez KR. Do healthy behaviors decline with greater acculturation? Implications for the Latino mortality paradox. Soc Sci Med 2005;61(6):1243–55.
7. Hunt LM, Schneider S, Comer B. Should "acculturation" be a variable in health research? A critical review of research on US Hispanics. Soc Sci Med 2004;59(5):973–86.
8. Marin G, Sabogal F, Marin BV, et al. Development of a short acculturation scale for Hispanics. Hisp J Behav Sci 1987;9(2):183–205.
9. Cuellar I, Arnold B, Maldonado R. Acculturation rating scale for Mexican Americans-II: a revision of the original ARSMA scale. Hisp J Behav Sci 1995;17(3):275–304.
10. Zong J, Batalova J. Frequently requested statistics on immigrants and immigration in the United States. Washington, DC: Migration Policy Institute; 2016. Available at: http://www.migrationpolicy.org/article/frequently-requested-statistics-immigrants-and-immigration-united-states#Top. Assessed August 24, 2016.
11. O'Hare W. The changing child population of the United States: analysis of data from the 2010 census. Baltimore, MD: The Annie E Foundation; 2016. Available at: http://www.aecf.org/m/resourcedoc/AECF-ChangingChildPopulation-2011-Full.pdf. Assessed August 24, 2016.
12. Child Trends. Immigrant children. 2014. Available at: http://www.childtrends.org/?indicators=immigrant-children. Accessed August 24, 2016.
13. Pew Research Center. Modern immigration wave brings 59 million to U.S., driving population growth and change through 2065 2015. Washington, DC: Pew Research Center. Available at: http://www.pewhispanic.org/files/2015/09/2015-09-28_modern-immigration-wave_REPORT.pdf. Assessed August 24, 2016.
14. Mejia GC, Kaufman JS, Corbie-Smith G, et al. A conceptual framework for Hispanic oral health care. J Public Health Dent 2008;68(1):1.
15. Scrimshaw SC. Our multicultural society: implications for pediatric dental practice. Pediatr Dent 2003;25(1):11–5.
16. Ng MW. Multicultural influences on child-rearing practices: implications for today's pediatric dentist. Pediatr Dent 2003;25(1):19–22.
17. Petti S. Why guidelines for early childhood caries prevention could be ineffective amongst children at high risk. J Dent 2010;38:946–55.
18. Patrick DL, Lee SY, Nucci M, et al. Reducing oral health disparities: a focus on social and cultural determinants. BMC Oral Health 2006;6(Suppl 1):S4.
19. Gao XL, McGrath C. A review on the oral health impacts of acculturation. J Immigr Minor Health 2011;13(2):202–13.
20. Horton S, Barker J. Stigmatized biologies: examining the cumulative effects of oral health disparities for Mexican American farmworker children. Med Anthropol Q 2010;24(2):199–219.

21. Farokhi MR, Cano SM, Bober-Moken IG, et al. Maternal acculturation could it impact oral health practices of Mexican-American mothers and their children? J Prim Care Community Health 2011;2(2):87–95.
22. Hoeft KS, Barker JC, Masterson EE. Urban Mexican-American mothers' beliefs about caries etiology in children. Community Dent Oral Epidemiol 2010;38(3): 244–55.
23. Tiwari T, Sharma T, Gutierrez K, et al. Learning about oral health knowledge & behavior in Latina mothers. Boston: IADR/AADR/CADR General Session & Exhibition; 2015.
24. Choi H. Cultural marginality: a concept analysis with implications for immigrant adolescents. Issues Compr Pediatr Nurs 2001;24(3):193–206.
25. Flores G, Tomany-Korman SC. Racial and ethnic disparities in medical and dental health, access to care, and use of services in US children. Pediatrics 2008; 121(2):e286–98.
26. Valencia A, Damiano P, Qian F, et al. Racial and ethnic disparities in utilization of dental services among children in Iowa: the Latino experience. Am J Public Health 2012;102(12):2352–9.
27. Cruz GD, Chen Y, Salazar CR, et al. The association of immigration and acculturation attributes with oral health among immigrants in New York City. Am J Public Health 2009;99(S2):S474–80.
28. Finlayson TL, Gansky SA, Shain SG, et al. Dental utilization by children in Hispanic agricultural worker families in California. J Dent Oral Craniofac Epidemiol 2014; 2(1–2):15.
29. Kim YO. Reducing disparities in dental care for low-income Hispanic children. J Health Care Poor Underserved 2005;16(3):431–43.
30. Mejia GC, Weintraub JA, Cheng NF, et al. Language and literacy relate to lack of children's dental sealant use. Community Dent Oral Epidemiol 2011;39(4): 318–24.
31. Telleen S, Kim R, Young O, et al. Access to oral health services for urban low-income Latino children: social ecological influences. J Public Health Dent 2012; 72(1):8–18.
32. Sanders AE. A Latino advantage in oral health-related quality of life is modified by nativity status. Soc Sci Med 2010;71(1):205–11.
33. Cubas YP, Orellana MF. The effect of acculturation in the concordance of oral health related quality of life in Latino children and their parents. Open Journal of Epidemiology 3: 95–104.
34. Acevedo-Garcia D, Bates LM. Latino health paradoxes: empirical evidence, explanations, future research, and implications. In: Rodriguez H, Saenz R, Menjivar C, editors. Latino/as in the United States: changing the face of America. New York: Springer. p. 101–13.
35. Hilton IV, Stephen S, Barker JC, et al. Cultural factors and children's oral health care: a qualitative study of carers of young children. Community Dent Oral Epidemiol 2007;35(6):429–38.
36. Wong D, Perez-Spiess S, Julliard K. Attitudes of Chinese parents toward the oral health of their children with caries: a qualitative study. Pediatr Dent 2005;27(6): 505–12.
37. Butani Y, Weintraub JA, Barker JC. Oral health-related cultural beliefs for four racial/ethnic groups: assessment of the literature. BMC Oral Health 2008;8(1):26.
38. Pham K, Barker JC, Walsh M. Oral health care of vietnamese adolescents: a qualitative study of perceptions and practices. J Dent Hyg 2015;89(6):397.

39. Cote S, Geltman P, Nunn M, et al. Dental caries of refugee children compared with US children. Pediatrics 2004;114(6):e733–40.
40. Obeng CS. Culture and dental health among African immigrant school-aged children in the United States. Health Educ 2007;107(4):343–50.
41. Graham MA, Tomar SL, Logan HL. Perceived social status, language and identified dental home among Hispanics in Florida. J Am Dent Assoc 2005;136(11):1572–82.
42. Mouradian WE, Berg JH, Somerman MJ. Addressing disparities through dental-medical collaborations, part 1. The role of cultural competency in health disparities: training of primary care medical practitioners in children's oral health. J Dent Educ 2003;67(8):860–8.
43. Riggs E, Gussy M, Gibbs L, et al. Hard to reach communities or hard to access services? Migrant mothers' experiences of dental services. Aust Dent J 2014;59(2):201–7.
44. De Jaimes FN, Batts F, Noguera C, et al. Implementation of language assessments for staff interpreters in community health centers. J Health Care Poor Underserved 2013;24(3):1002–9.
45. Jacobs EA, Lauderdale DS, Meltzer D, et al. Impact of interpreter services on delivery of health care to limited–English-proficient patients. J Gen Intern Med 2001;16(7):468–74.
46. Mariño R, Morgan M, Hopcraft M. Transcultural dental training: addressing the oral health care needs of people from culturally diverse backgrounds. Community Dent Oral Epidemiol 2012;40(s2):134–40.
47. Garcia RI, Cadoret CA, Henshaw M. Multicultural issues in oral health. Dent Clin North Am 2008;52:319–32.
48. Formicola AJ, Stavisky J, Lewy R. Cultural competency: dentistry and medicine learning from one another. J Dent Educ 2003;67(8):869–75.
49. Valachovic RW. Current demographics and future trends of the dentist workforce 2009. In US Oral Health Workforce in the Coming Decade: A Workshop. Available at: http://www.nationalacademies.org/hmd/~/media/Files/Activity%20Files/Workforce/oralhealthworkforce/2009-Feb-09/1%20-%20Valachovic.ashx. Assessed August 24, 2016.
50. US Department of Health and Human Services. Sex, race, and ethnic diversity of US health occupations 2010-2012. Available at: http://bhpr.hrsa.gov/healthworkforce/supplydemand/usworkforce/diversityushealthoccupations.pdf. Accessed August 1, 2016.
51. Brick C, McCully SN, Updegraff JA, et al. Impact of cultural exposure and message framing on oral health behavior exploring the role of message memory. Med Decis Making 2016;36(7):834–43.
52. Nicol P, Al-Hanbali A, King N, et al. Informing a culturally appropriate approach to oral health and dental care for pre-school refugee children: a community participatory study. BMC Oral Health 2014;14(1):1.
53. Tiwari T, Sharma T, Harper M, et al. Community based participatory research to reduce oral health disparities in American Indian children. J Fam Med 2015;2(3):1028.
54. Tiwari T, Casciello A, Gansky SA, et al. Recruitment for health disparities preventive intervention trials: the early childhood caries collaborating centers. Prev Chronic Dis 2014;11:E133.
55. Garcia RI, Tiwari T, Ramos-Gomez F, et al. Retention Strategies for health disparities preventive trials: findings from the early childhood caries collaborating centers. J Public Health Dent 2017;77(1):63–77.

56. Ramos-Gomez FJ, Gansky SA, Featherstone JD, et al. Mother and youth access (MAYA) maternal chlorhexidine, counselling and pediatric fluoride varnish randomized clinical trial to prevent early childhood caries. Int J Paediatr Dent 2012;22:169–79.
57. Harrison RL, Wong T. An oral health promotion program for an urban minority population of preschool children. Community Dent Oral Epidemiol 2003;31(5): 392–9.
58. Weinstein P, Harrison R, Benton T. Motivating parents to prevent caries in their young children: one-year findings. J Am Dent Assoc 2004;135(6):731–8.
59. Hoeft KS, Barker JC, Shiboski S, et al. Effectiveness evaluation of Contra Caries Oral Health Education Program for improving Spanish-speaking parents' preventive oral health knowledge and behaviors for their young children. Community Dent Oral Epidemiol 2016;44(6):564–76.
60. Albino J, Tiwari T. Preventing childhood caries a review of recent behavioral research. J Dent Res 2016;95:35–42.
61. Biordi DL, Heitzer M, Mundy E, et al. Improving access and provision of preventive oral health care for very young, poor, and low-income children through a new interdisciplinary partnership. Am J Public Health 2015;105(S2):e23–9.
62. Melvin CS. A collaborative community-based oral care program for school-age children. Clin Nurse Spec 2006;20(1):18–22.
63. Crall JJ, Illum J, Martinez A, et al. An innovative project breaks down barriers to oral health care for vulnerable young children in Los Angeles county. Policy Brief UCLA Cent Health Policy Res 2016;(PB2016–5):1–8.

Interventions Focusing on Children with Special Health Care Needs

Paul Glassman, DDS, MA, MBA

KEYWORDS

- Children with special health care needs ● Children with special needs ● Oral health
- Interventions

KEY POINTS

- Children with special health care needs (CSHCN) refers to "those who have or are at increased risk for a chronic physical, developmental, behavioral, or emotional condition and who also require health and related services of a type or amount beyond that required by children generally."
- CSHCN can be classified by age, sex, poverty status, race/ethnicity, and impact of their condition on daily activity, including dental care utilization.
- It is difficult to make generalizable dental care recommendations for CSHCN because there is a wide variety of conditions that are encompassed by the term CSHCN and the subsequent difficulty producing recommendations that apply across this spectrum. The term "children with special needs" is suggested when considering clinical care and guidelines.

CHILDREN WITH SPECIAL HEALTH CARE NEEDS

The term "children with special health care needs" (CSHCN) has various definitions in the literature. One definition commonly cited is "those who have or are at increased risk for a chronic physical, developmental, behavioral, or emotional condition and who also require health and related services of a type or amount beyond that required by children generally."[1–3] A National Survey of Children with Special Health Care Needs (NS-CSHCN) was conducted 3 times between 2001 and 2010. It was designed to take a close look at the health and functional status of CSHCNs in the United States; their physical, emotional, and behavioral health; along with critical information on access to quality health care, care coordination of services, access to a medical home, transition services for youth, and the impact of chronic condition(s) on the child's family.[4] In the future, this survey will be combined with National Survey on Children's Health.[5]

Disclosures: The author has no commercial or financial interests to disclose.
University of the Pacific Arthur A. Dugoni School of Dentistry, 155 5th Street, San Francisco, California 94904, USA
E-mail address: pglassman@pacific.edu

Dent Clin N Am 61 (2017) 565–576
http://dx.doi.org/10.1016/j.cden.2017.02.007
dental.theclinics.com

Results of the last NS-CSHCN was published in 2013 as a Chartbook for 2009 to 2010. It uses a short CSHCN Screener designed to identify CSHCN in household surveys.[6,7] Based on that tool, it was reported that 15.1% of children younger than 18, or approximately 11.2 million children, were estimated to have special health care needs. Overall, 23% of US households with children had at least 1 child with special health care needs. The CSHCN Screener, as used in the NS-CSHCN, contains screening questions with 5 major components. In addition to the presence of a condition that has lasted or is expected to last at least 1 year, the respondent must report at least 1 of the following consequences for the child:

- The use of or need for prescription medication
- The use of or need for more medical care, mental health services, or education services than other children of the same age
- An ongoing emotional, behavioral, or developmental problem that requires treatment or counseling
- A limitation in the child's ability to do the things that most children of the same age do
- The use of or need for special therapy, such as physical, occupational, or speech therapy.

As illustrated in **Fig. 1**, of these 5 qualifying criteria, the need for prescription medication is by far the most common, reported by more than three-fourths of CSHCN. The

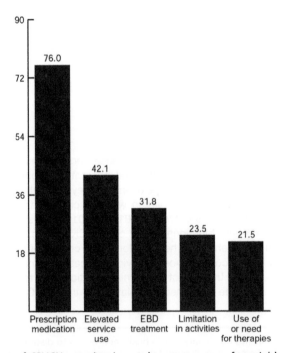

Fig. 1. Percentage of CSHCN experiencing each consequence of special health care needs. (*From* US Department of Health and Human Services, Health Resources and Services Administration, Maternal and Child Health Bureau. The National Survey of Children with Special Health Care Needs Chartbook 2009–2010. Rockville (MD): US Department of Health and Human Services; 2013. Available at: http://mchb.hrsa.gov/cshcn0910/more/pdf/nscshcn0910.pdf. Accessed October 15, 2016; with permission.)

next most frequently reported consequence is the use of or need for extra medical, mental health, or educational services (42.1% of CSHCN), followed by need for or use of services for ongoing emotional, behavioral, or developmental problems (31.8%), limitation in activities (23.5%), and the use of specialized therapies (21.5%).

The NS-CSHCN 2009 to 2010 also reported on the prevalence of CSHCN by age, sex, poverty status, race/ethnicity, and other characteristics. **Figs. 2–5** illustrate some of these findings.

IMPACT OF SPECIAL HEALTH CARE CONDITIONS

Although the data presented previously is illustrative of the number of children who meet the definition of CSHCN, it does not describe the functional consequences of these conditions on the child. The NS-CSHCN asked about the impact of these conditions on the child's daily activities. **Figs. 6–8** illustrate the impact of these conditions on daily activities by poverty status, race/ethnicity, and primary language.

In addition to describing the percentage of CSHCN that had impacts on daily activities, the NS-CSHCN also reported on the percentage of children with various categories of functional difficulties. These included limitations in "bodily function," which was defined as breathing or respiration, swallowing or digestion, blood circulation, chronic physical pain including headaches, seeing even when wearing glasses or contacts, and hearing even when using a hearing aid. It also included limitations in "participating in any activity" which was defined as "self-care, coordination or moving around, using hands, learning, understanding or paying attention, speaking, communicating or being understood." Finally, it included emotional or behavioral limitations for children 10 months to 17 years old. The relative percentages of these types of difficulties are illustrated in **Fig. 8**.

The NS-CSHCN also reported on other consequences of children's conditions. It was reported that the average child misses 3 days of school, whereas the average

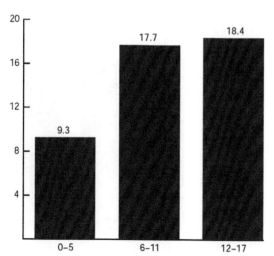

Fig. 2. Percentage of CSHCN by age. (*From* US Department of Health and Human Services, Health Resources and Services Administration, Maternal and Child Health Bureau. The National Survey of Children with Special Health Care Needs Chartbook 2009–2010. Rockville (MD): US Department of Health and Human Services; 2013. Available at: http://mchb.hrsa.gov/cshcn0910/more/pdf/nscshcn0910.pdf. Accessed October 15, 2016; with permission.)

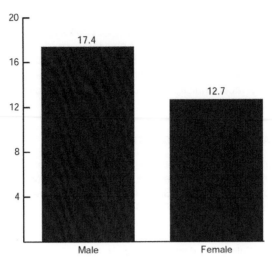

Fig. 3. Percentage of CSHCN by sex. (*From* US Department of Health and Human Services, Health Resources and Services Administration, Maternal and Child Health Bureau. The National Survey of Children with Special Health Care Needs Chartbook 2009–2010. Rockville (MD): US Department of Health and Human Services; 2013. Available at: http://mchb.hrsa. gov/cshcn0910/more/pdf/nscshcn0910.pdf. Accessed October 15, 2016; with permission.)

CSHCN misses 6.7 days. However, some children missed much more school with 22% of the lowest income CSHCN missing 11 days or more of school annually.

Although the NS-CSHCN is the most comprehensive data set available about CSHCN, there are many other publications that provide information about these

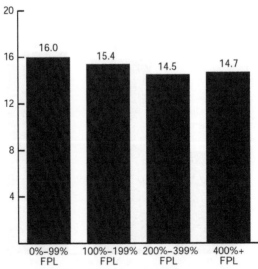

Fig. 4. Percent of CSHCN by poverty status. (*From* US Department of Health and Human Services, Health Resources and Services Administration, Maternal and Child Health Bureau. The National Survey of Children with Special Health Care Needs Chartbook 2009–2010. Rockville (MD): US Department of Health and Human Services; 2013. Available at: http://mchb.hrsa. gov/cshcn0910/more/pdf/nscshcn0910.pdf. Accessed October 15, 2016; with permission.)

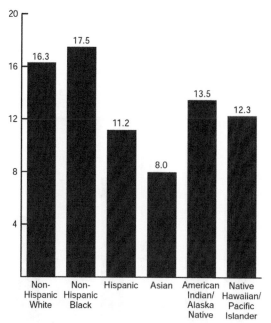

Fig. 5. Percentage of CSHCN by race/ethnicity. (*From* US Department of Health and Human Services, Health Resources and Services Administration, Maternal and Child Health Bureau. The National Survey of Children with Special Health Care Needs Chartbook 2009–2010. Rockville (MD): US Department of Health and Human Services; 2013. Available at: http://mchb.hrsa.gov/cshcn0910/more/pdf/nscshcn0910.pdf. Accessed October 15, 2016; with permission.)

children and, in particular, their oral health status. The Institute of Medicine (IOM), in the 2011 report on *Improving Access to Oral Health Care for Vulnerable and Underserved Populations*, pointed out that people with special health care needs (SHCN) are among the population groups in the United States who are not well served by the oral health care system.[8] The IOM reported that most, although not all, studies indicate that the overall prevalence of dental caries in people with SHCN is either the same as the general population or slightly lower. However, available data indicate that people with SHCN suffer disproportionately from periodontal disease and edentulism, have more untreated dental caries, poorer oral hygiene, and receive less care than the general population.

A 2012 publication analyzed the use of CSHCN Screener tool to predict the risk for poor oral health and unmet dental needs.[9] The investigators found that the number of positive CSHCN Screener criteria was independently associated with various parent-perceived poorer oral health outcomes in children. CSHCN who met 4 or 5 screener criteria had 4 and 4.5 times, respectively, the odds of having fair-poor condition of teeth and bleeding gums relative to non-CSHCN. They also had 87% higher odds for parent-perceived toothache and 2 and 2.5 times the odds of having recent broken teeth and unmet dental care needs relative to non-CSHCN, respectively.

There is long-standing evidence that CSHCN have more unmet dental needs than children who do not.[10] They also use more dental care services, but those services are more likely to be nonpreventive services. It is likely that dental care services were more apt to be received after disease had developed rather than earlier when disease needing treatment could have been prevented.

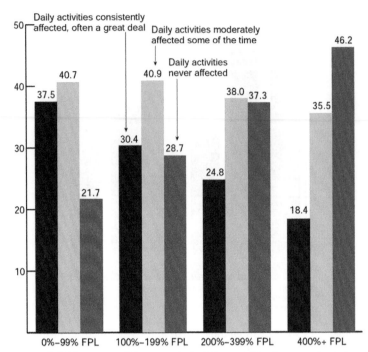

Fig. 6. Impact of children's conditions on their daily activities by poverty status. (*From* US Department of Health and Human Services, Health Resources and Services Administration, Maternal and Child Health Bureau. The National Survey of Children with Special Health Care Needs Chartbook 2009–2010. Rockville (MD): US Department of Health and Human Services; 2013. Available at: http://mchb.hrsa.gov/cshcn0910/more/pdf/nscshcn0910.pdf. Accessed October 15, 2016; with permission.)

INTERVENTIONS

The data presented previously clearly indicate that there are large numbers of children who meet the definition of CSHCN. The data also indicate that those in lower income groups and racial and ethnic minorities face greater challenges receiving dental care as is the case with other population groups and conditions.[8] However, it is not clear whether these results are directly related to the conditions these children have or whether they are a result of the time, attention, money, or other resources expended by parents because of the child's condition. It follows that one reason that CSHCN have more unmet dental needs is because of the burden on their parents related to their SHCN. A 2013 analysis was performed on the relation between caregiver burden and preventive dental care for CSHCN.[11] When the child's health condition impacted work, time spent on health management, and finances, the use of preventive dental care decreased. The investigators recommended that interventions to improve the oral health of CSHCN should include strategies to reduce caregiver burden, especially within socioeconomically vulnerable families.

Although the term CSHCN is useful to define populations for funding and research purposes, it is less useful when considering evidence and guidelines for "interventions" or clinical care. This is because it includes children with many different conditions and situations. It also includes children with conditions that are unrelated to the child's ability to receive dental care and unrelated to the development or

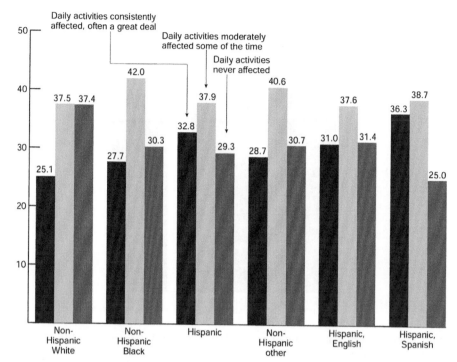

Fig. 7. Impact of CSHCN's conditions on their daily activities by race/ethnicity and primary language. (*From* US Department of Health and Human Services, Health Resources and Services Administration, Maternal and Child Health Bureau. The National Survey of Children with Special Health Care Needs Chartbook 2009–2010. Rockville (MD): US Department of Health and Human Services; 2013. Available at: http://mchb.hrsa.gov/cshcn0910/more/pdf/nscshcn0910.pdf. Accessed October 15, 2016; with permission.)

exacerbation of dental disease. Other classification terms related to CSHCN include "children with special needs," "children with disabilities," and "children with complex conditions."[12–14] Although these terms do not have generally agreed on precise definitions, they are widely used and useful in describing populations that present challenges in providing oral health services. For the purpose of the remainder of this article, the terms "children with special needs," will be used along with CSHCN. A broad definition of these terms is used: children who have difficulty accessing or receiving dental services because of complicated medical, physical, social, or psychological conditions.[15]

Given the wide variety of conditions encompassed by CSHCN or children with special needs, there are no standard interventions that apply across all these conditions. The primary issue in creating and maintaining oral health for children in these categories is performing a thorough assessment of their conditions and situations and planning and providing customized oral health services that consider the findings. Customized services include what is done, where it is done, by whom, and in what time sequence.[16]

CHALLENGES IN PROVIDING ORAL HEALTH CARE FOR PEOPLE WITH SPECIAL NEEDS

There are numerous challenges in providing oral health services for people with special needs that go beyond the normal considerations for other populations. First, there

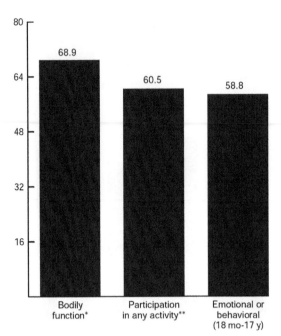

Fig. 8. Types of functional difficulties among CSHCN. (*From* US Department of Health and Human Services, Health Resources and Services Administration, Maternal and Child Health Bureau. The National Survey of Children with Special Health Care Needs Chartbook 2009–2010. Rockville (MD): US Department of Health and Human Services; 2013. Available at: http://mchb.hrsa.gov/cshcn0910/more/pdf/nscshcn0910.pdf. Accessed October 15, 2016; with permission.)

is a need to understand and to be prepared to work with people with a wide variety of general health conditions. Although oral health professionals do not need to have complete knowledge of every general health condition with which their patients present, it is essential that they have the knowledge and experience to gather and apply the information they need. This implies the training and ability to function in health care teams and get consultations from physicians, social workers, and other general and social service professionals.

There is also a need for oral health professionals to understand the social service systems that operate in their community and the social context in which oral health services take place. They need to understand community living arrangements, social service agencies, and advocacy organizations operating in their community. They also need to understand the appropriate use of language when interacting with individuals with special needs and their caregivers. There is a growing movement advocating the use of "People First" language.[17–20] This language emphasizes that disability is a part of the human condition and all people want to be described by their abilities rather than labeled by their disabilities. An oral health professional who does not understand this language and refers to people he treats as "the handicapped patients I see" risks alienating the individual, the individual caregiver, and those advocating for full inclusion in our society. An example of the use of People First language is to refer to "people with disabilities" rather the "the disabled." Although these phrases might seem similar, the former phrase indicates that this is a group that has a particular condition. It implies that the group has other characteristics as well, collectively and individually.

The latter phrase implies that the disability is the prime and even only characteristic that needs to be considered for this group.

Oral health professionals also need to understand the extraordinary vulnerability of people with special needs to abuse and neglect in our society.[21,22] They need to understand how to recognize abuse and neglect and their role as mandated reporters. Oral health providers are health professionals, and as a part of the health care team they may find that their patients are depressed, suicidal, or unable to cope with various living challenges. They have an obligation to intervene, provide basic diagnosis and counseling, and make appropriate referrals for follow-up of these situations.

Oral health professionals also need to understand how to support prevention of oral diseases in people with various disabilities. There are special challenges presented by working with someone in whom communication and even procedures need to be performed by a third person, the caregiver. Some people have limited physical ability to perform oral hygiene procedures and "partial participation" programs need to be designed and carried out. This term refers to having the individual do as much as he or she is able to, but having a caregiver ensure that needed prevention procedures are completed. There are numerous informational, physical, behavioral obstacles to be addressed. These are described in detail in a caregiver training package titled "Overcoming Obstacles to Dental Health," a training package for caregivers of people with disabilities.[23] In addition to this package, there is a large literature that describes the challenges and techniques for helping people with special needs prevent oral diseases.[24–27]

The American Academy of Pediatric Dentistry has summarized conditions and recommendations for management of dental patients with SHCN.[28] However a review of the guidelines reveals that they are focused on children needing behavior support to receive dental care and basically the same guidelines as would be recommended for children without SHCN. Again, this is inevitable given the wide variety of conditions that are encompassed by the term CSHCN and the subsequent difficulty producing recommendations that apply across this spectrum.

Some oral health providers have requested a recipe for "what to do" for people with a specific condition. As indicated here, this is not possible because of the wide variety of factors that may or may not be present in multiple individuals, all of whom have that specific condition. A customized plan needs to be based on gathering, analyzing, synthesizing, and drawing conclusions that are combined into a customized plan.[29] Factors to be considered include the following:

- General health condition(s)
- Medical prognosis
- Functional reserve
- Degree of dependence
- Communication ability
- Ability to have dental care in a dental office
- Caregiver participation in daily mouth care activities and facilitation of dental treatment
- Social support system
- Financial resources
- Dental condition(s)
- Dental prognosis
- Individual's expectations and desires

It is only when these factors are understood and carefully considered that a customized plan can be developed that is the optimum plan for that individual.

SUMMARY AND FUTURE RESEARCH

The term CSHCN encompasses a wide variety of conditions. There are data on the number of children who meet the condition in this classification scheme, the consequences of their conditions, and the impact of these conditions in general on daily activities. However, most of these data are descriptive of the population and other than the recommendation to reduce caregiver burden, do not tie specific qualifying conditions to specific clinical care guidelines.

To develop an approach and plan for a single individual, data need to be gathered, and analyzed, synthesized, and conclusions drawn about many factors related to the individuals' health and social circumstances.

When considering interventions, a broader definition of children with special needs is suggested in this article, along with a focus on developing specific treatment recommendations based on a thorough data-gathering process and developing customized recommendations for the child based on his or her unique circumstances. An area for future research is increasing the understanding of the relationship between customized recommendations and the underlying SHCN.

REFERENCES

1. U.S. Department of Health and Human Services, Health Resources and Services Administration, Maternal and Child Health Bureau. The national survey of children with special health care needs Chartbook 2009–2010. Rockville (MD): U.S. Department of Health and Human Services; 2013. Available at: http://mchb.hrsa.gov/cshcn0910/more/pdf/nscshcn0910.pdf. Accessed October 15, 2016.
2. U.S. Department of Health and Human Services. Healthcare Emergency Preparedness Information Gateway. Supporting children with special healthcare needs. Available at: https://asprtracie.hhs.gov/technical-resources/MasterSearch?qt=supporting+children+with+special+healthcare+needs&page=1 and https://asprtracie.hhs.gov/documents/supportingcshcnmatrix.pdf. Accessed October 15, 2016.
3. McPherson M, Arango P, Fox H, et al. A new definition of children with special health care needs. Pediatrics 1998;102(1):137–40.
4. CDC. National Center for Health Statistics. Child and Adolescent Health Measurement Initiative. Child and Adolescent Health. National Survey of Children with Special Health. Available at: http://www.childhealthdata.org/learn/NS-CSHCN. Accessed October 15, 2016.
5. HRSA. MCHB. National Survey Publications and Chartbooks. Available at: http://mchb.hrsa.gov/data-research-epidemiology/research-epidemiology/national-survey-publications-and-chartbooks. Accessed on October 15, 2016.
6. HHS. HRSA. MCHB. The National Survey of Children with Special Health Care Needs (NS-CSHCN) Chartbook 2009-2010. 2013. Available at: http://mchb.hrsa.gov/cshcn0910/more/pdf/nscshcn0910.pdf. Accessed October 15, 2016.
7. Bethell C, Read D, Stein RE, et al. Identifying children with special health care needs: development and evaluation of a short screening instrument. Ambul Pediatr 2002;2(1):38–48.
8. IOM (Institute of Medicine), NRC (National Research Council). Improving access to oral health care for vulnerable and underserved populations. Washington, DC: The National Academies Press; 2011.
9. Iida H, Lewis CW. Utility of a summative scale based on the children with special health care needs (CSHCN) screener to identify CSHCN with special dental care needs. Matern Child Health J 2012;16:1164–72.

10. Lisa H, Lewis C, Zhou C, et al. Dental care needs, use and expenditures among U.S. children with and without special health care needs. J Am Dent Assoc 2010; 141(1):79–88.
11. Chi DL, McManus BM, Carle AC. Caregiver burden and preventive dental care use for us children with special health care needs: a stratified analysis based on functional limitation. Matern Child Health J 2014;18:882–90.
12. Waldman HB, Perlman SP, Waldman HB, et al. Children with special health care needs: results of a national survey. J Dent Child 2006;73(1):57–62.
13. U.S. Department of Health and Human Services. Oral health in America: a report of the surgeon general. Rockville (MD): U.S. Department of Health and Human Services; National Institute of Dental and Craniofacial Research; National Institutes of Health; 2000.
14. Glassman P, Henderson T, Helgeson M, et al. Consensus statement: oral health for people with special needs: consensus statement on implications and recommendations for the dental profession. J Calif Dent Assoc 2005; 33(8):619–23.
15. Glassman P, Anderson M, Jacobsen P, et al. Practical protocols for the prevention of dental disease in community settings for people with special needs: the protocols. Spec Care Dentist 2003;23(5):86–90.
16. Glassman P, Subar P. Improving and maintaining oral health for people with special needs. Dent Clin North Am 2008;52:447–61.
17. CDC. Communicating with and about people with disabilities. Available at: https://www.cdc.gov/ncbddd/disabilityandhealth/pdf/disabilityposter_photos.pdf. Accessed October 15, 2016.
18. Snow K. People first language. Available at: http://www.disabilityisnatural.com/peoplefirstlanguage.htm. Accessed September 1, 2007.
19. West Virginians with Developmental Disabilities. People First Language. Available at: http://www.wvddc.org/people_first.html. Accessed September 1, 2007.
20. The Life Span Institute. Guidelines for reporting and writing about people with disabilities. Available at: http://www.lsi.ku.edu/lsi/internal/guidelines.html. Accessed September 1, 2007.
21. Glassman P, Chavez E, Hawks D. Abuse and neglect of elderly individuals: guidelines for oral health professionals. J Calif Dent Assoc 2004;32(4):232–335.
22. Glassman P, Miller C, Ingraham R, et al. The extraordinary vulnerability of people with disabilities: guidelines for oral health professionals. J Calif Dent Assoc 2004; 32(5):379–86.
23. Miller C, Glassman P, Wozniak T, et al. Overcoming obstacles to dental health: a training program for caregivers of people with disabilities. 4th edition. 1998.
24. Glassman P, Miller C. Dental disease prevention and people with special needs. CDA J 2003;31(2):149–60.
25. Glassman P, Anderson M, Jacobsen P, et al. Practical protocols for the prevention of dental disease in community settings for people with special needs: the protocols. Spec Care Dentist 2003;23(5):160–4.
26. Glassman P, Miller C. Preventing dental disease for people with special needs: the need for practical preventive protocols for use in community settings. Spec Care Dentist 2003;23(5):165–7.
27. Glassman P, Miller C. Effect of preventive dentistry training program for caregivers in community facilities on caregiver and client behavior and client oral hygiene. NY State Dent J 2006;72(2):38–46.

28. AAPD. Guideline on management of dental patients with special health care needs. 2012. Available at: http://www.aapd.org/media/policies_guidelines/g_ shcn.pdf. Accessed October 15, 2016.

29. Glassman P, Subar P. Planning dental treatment for people with special needs. Dent Clin North Am 2009;53(2):195–205.

Pediatric Workforce Issues

Elizabeth Mertz, PhD, MA[a],*, Joanne Spetz, PhD[b],
Jean Moore, DrPH, MSN[c]

KEYWORDS

- Health personnel • Pediatric dentistry • Allied health personnel
- Dental care for children • Dental care delivery

KEY POINTS

- There are many new workforce models being deployed to address children's oral health.
- Evaluations of these models are variable, showing safety and effectiveness but rarely impact on health outcomes.
- Health professions regulatory barriers exist that restrict the ability to fully deploy new models.

INTRODUCTION

According to the US Surgeon General, dental disease is among the most prevalent health conditions for children, and large disparities in oral health status and access to oral health services exist among children in the United State.[1] In 2003, the *National Call to Action to Promote Oral Health* outlined the need to increase the diversity, capacity, and flexibility of the dental workforce in order to better meet children's oral health needs and reduce disparities.[2] Assessing progress toward the *Call to Action*, in 2009 the authors found only modest gains in workforce strategies focused on pediatric patients, and major challenges remaining.[3] In 2009 the Institute of Medicine held a workshop on the sufficiency of the oral health workforce for the coming decade, which outlined the status of the dental workforce, and highlighted for the first time the multitude of new workforce models being proposed and tried.[4] A special issue of the *Journal of Public Health Dentistry* entirely focused on the contributions of workforce innovations to delivery system redesign followed, with one of the key messages being that workforce design should be tied directly to meeting the patient care needs, with special attention to reducing disparities in oral health care, and in oral health.[5] As

Disclosures: The authors have nothing to disclose.
[a] Preventive and Restorative Dental Sciences, Healthforce Center, University of California, San Francisco, 3333 California Street, Suite 410, San Francisco, CA 94143, USA; [b] Philip R. Lee Institute for Health Policy Studies, Healthforce Center, University of California, San Francisco, 3333 California Street, Suite 265, San Francisco, CA 94143, USA; [c] Center for Health Workforce Studies, School of Public Health, University at Albany, State University of New York, 1 University Place, Suite 220, Rensselaer, NY 12144, USA
* Corresponding author.
E-mail address: Elizabeth.mertz@ucsf.edu

http://dx.doi.org/10.1016/j.cden.2017.02.004
0011-8532/17/© 2017 Elsevier Inc. All rights reserved.

dental.theclinics.com

2017 begins, progress has been documented in children's use of care primarily because of improvements in coverage through Medicaid, the Children's Health Insurance Program (CHIP), and the Affordable Care Act (ACA).[6,7] This article updates and synthesizes the evidence on clinical pediatric workforce models and discusses future directions and implications for health policy.

METHODOLOGY

This study reviews journal publications, reports, and issue briefs regarding evidence-based approaches to enhancing the workforce available to address children's oral health. The article organizes the findings into (1) new models in the dental field, including existing and new providers; and (2) workforce models outside the dental field.[3] Interdisciplinary models constitute a growing area of innovation in workforce configurations (see Edelstein BL: Pediatric Dental-Focused Inter-Professional Interventions: Rethinking Early Childhood Oral Health Management, in this issue). Case studies from programs of particular interest are provided to illustrate real world applications from ongoing pilots or programs.

RESULTS
The Traditional Dental Team

The core of pediatric dental care lies with the traditional team of dentists, hygienists, and dental assistants. With the opening of 12 new US dental schools and expansion of enrollment from 4300 to 5900 dentists per year, the overall supply of dentists is projected to increase.[8] However, geographic shortages, a lack of diversity, and a lack of participation in Medicaid persist and affect the availability of dental care for children, particularly in rural, high-minority, and low-income areas.[9] This pattern is exacerbated among pediatric dentists, who tend to concentrate in higher-income areas despite the burden of complex disease being borne by disadvantaged children.[10] The need for future pediatric dentists ready and willing to treat a diverse patient pool has led to changes in the pediatric residency curriculum that incorporate a greater focus on patients who are low income, minority, and have special care needs.[11] In addition, residencies in general dentistry (Advanced Education in General Dentistry/General Practice Residency) are increasingly providing clinical training in pediatric dental care.[12] First-year enrollment in pediatric dental residencies has increased from 292 in 2004 to 436 in 2014, and the number of programs increased from 65 to 77 during that time frame, but the specialty remains a small portion of the dental workforce.[13]

General dentists continue to provide most of the care for children. Predoctoral training programs are challenged in adequately preparing general dentists to treat children, in part because of the school dental clinic population mix being composed primarily of adults. Therefore, general dentists are often reluctant to treat children less than 3 years of age despite increasing practitioner recognition that children should have their first dental visit by age one.[14,15] General dentists are more willing to see young children who are low caries risk or for prevention than children who are high risk or need restorative treatment.[16–19] Recommendations have been made to change the Commission on Dental Accreditation (CODA) accreditation standards for dental schools to strengthen training in oral health care for young children, but this has not been enacted.[20] In recognition of this need for improved pediatric skills for general dentists, many states have initiated trainings for providers specifically on reaching young children, but overall data on trends are not available.[21–25]

Dental hygienists are important members of the oral health team and their roles in pediatric care have been expanding. Hygienists are often the first point of contact, providing evaluation and assessment of patients' oral health status, oral health education and preventive care, and referral to dental providers for necessary treatment services. Hygienists increasingly are providing community outreach to underserved populations, serving as case finders and care managers who refer for dental treatment services and encourage establishment of dental homes[26,27] (see the case studies presented later). Dental hygiene scope of practice has evolved over time, with hygienists in many states practicing more autonomously than they had previously, particularly in public health settings such as schools, nursing homes, and correctional facilities. However, scope of practice parameters in some states limit the ability of hygienists to effectively provide services in the community. Allowing hygienists to work to the full extent of their professional competence facilitates access to services, especially for underserved populations.[28] An assessment of dental hygiene scope of practice across states found a positive correlation between broader dental hygiene scope of practice and better oral health outcomes.[28,29]

Dental assistants are key members of the oral health workforce team, performing both clinical and administrative duties under the supervision of a dentist. In addition to directly assisting dentists with oral examinations and dental procedures, dental assistants perform several independent tasks, including preparing patients for treatment, arranging and sterilizing instruments, and educating patients about general and postoperative oral health care. Dental assistants also act in administrative capacities, including scheduling appointments, maintaining patient records, and billing for treatment services. However, there is variability across states in the required education and training to enter the workforce as a dental assistant, in the titles used to describe the workforce, and in the legally allowed functions. Many states now recognize expanded function dental assistants. Expanded functions permitted to appropriately trained individuals include coronal polishing, sealant and/or fluoride applications, and topical anesthetic application, as well as expanded restorative and orthodontic functions. It is unclear how much this changes clinical pediatric practice, and one study found that expanded function assistants do not use this function most of the time.[30] Recent research suggests that dental assistants, especially expanded function dental assistants, contribute to improved clinical efficiency and increased access to oral health services.[31]

Expanding the Dental Team

In response to the limitations of the current dental team's capacity to address pediatric dental care needs there has been an expansion into new roles, to fill gaps in providers available for treatment as well as to improve access and prevention.

Dental therapists have been used across the world by many countries as part of the health care team, with a primary focus on children.[32] In 2003, the Alaska Native Tribal Health Consortium (ANTHC) was the first to implement the use of dental therapists.[33] Since then, advocates of this role have successfully changed policy to allow dental therapists to practice in Minnesota, Maine, and Vermont, whereas Washington and Oregon have tribal access authorized and statewide use under consideration and 9 more states are actively investigating their use.[34,35] Dental therapist have the ability to do restorative and other dental procedures normally restricted to dentists. Each state has defined the role slightly differently, and states that recognize dental therapist seem to be leaning toward a combined hygiene-therapy model. In 2016 the CODA adopted standards for dental therapy education programs and put a process in place for accrediting them. The research on impacts of dental therapists on oral health access and outcomes is emerging and has generally found them to be safe and effective practitioners.[36] For example, dental therapists in Alaska were able to treat children with the same clinical effectiveness as dentists.[37] In addition, dental therapists have been shown to be profitable in the clinical enterprise, allowing dentists to focus on more complex cases, and may be used in school-based care for children.[38,39] The primary dental health aide role in Alaska, which is part of the 4-step dental health aide cadre in ANTHC, is discussed later.

The community dental health coordinator (CDHC) was designed to function much like a community health worker with an oral health focus. The CDHC concept is being piloted in 8 states and, as of 2014, the project has 34 graduates who are serving in 26 communities in Arizona, California, Montana, Minnesota, Oklahoma, Pennsylvania, Texas, and Wisconsin.[40] CDHCs are trained to provide community education about oral health, case finding, patient navigation, and patient engagement services using motivational interviewing techniques. In a series of case studies on oral health integration with primary care, one clinic used a CDHC who was also a licensed dental hygienist and was additionally qualified as a public health dental hygiene practitioner (PHDHP) in Pennsylvania. The CDHC/PHDHP was active in the community providing oral health education at community events, schools, Head Start programs, and other settings. In addition, she was working in primary care practices affiliated with the clinic providing dental hygiene assessment and prophylactic services and navigating new patients to the main dental clinic for treatment services.[31] Other research has found that CDHCs have reduced no-show visits and increased clinic productivity.[41]

Expanding the Oral Health Team

In 2003 the American Academy of Pediatrics affirmed its critical role by establishing a policy that pediatricians should know how to do risk assessments and refer high-risk children to a dental home.[42] The Into the Mouths of Babes project in North Carolina's Medicaid program showed the effectiveness of fluoride varnish applications by physicians in reducing caries treatment needs and this is now a widely covered benefit.[43,44] Studies have shown that application of fluoride varnish by primary care providers is just as effective in reducing caries as prevention by dental providers, and reimbursing primary care providers for this has increased the uptake of this treatment.[45–47] Most pediatricians now agree that they should examine their patients' mouths and discuss oral hygiene with families, but only about half report doing it. Further, although they know the benefit of fluoride varnish, few physicians regularly apply it for their patients, citing barriers including lack of training and reimbursement.[48,49] By 2011, 42 states had adopted a policy to support preventive dentistry initiatives for physicians.[50] Two examples of these types of initiatives are discussed later.

In the primary care setting, nurse practitioners and physician assistants (PAs) are also playing an increasing role in oral care for children. For example, in one study a nurse-dietitian team was used to provide preventive care and referrals, increasing access and acceptance of fluoride varnish.[51] This example is a model for allied health professionals to integrate an oral health screen, fluoride varnish, anticipatory guidance, and dental referrals.[52] Further, obstetricians and gynecologists are becoming more educated on the importance of improving the oral health literacy of pregnant women, which substantially influences the knowledge and behaviors of pregnant women regarding the importance of oral health.[53]

A 2013 survey of directors of PA education programs found that more than 70% of respondent programs had integrated oral health topics into the core content of their PA curricula.[54] However, whether training in oral health in PA education programs translates into screening and assessment of patients' oral health statuses in clinical practice remains unclear. A 2013 survey of PAs conducted by the American Association of Physician Assistants identified several key barriers to the effective integration of oral health competency into practice.[55] For example, completion of oral examinations or fluoride varnish by PAs is not as widely reimbursable as when completed by nurses or physicians.[56] However, a low survey response rate limits the ability to generalize from these results. The Oral Health Workforce Research Center (OHWRC) conducted a sample survey of PAs to learn more about the integration of oral health assessment and screening into their clinical practices. The study found that PAs trained in oral health as part of their basic PA education program were nearly 3 times as likely to conduct oral health screenings, compared to those who did not receive training.[57]

In addition, programs that use community health workers who incorporate oral health into their work have been shown to increase knowledge of oral health among their clients and increase efficiencies in dental clinics.[58–60] The coordination of care outside what is provided in the dental office remains challenging across the dental-medical divide.[61,62]

A 2014 HRSA-sponsored report, *Integration of Oral Health and Primary Care Practice*, described core oral health clinical competencies for frontline primary care clinicians and outlined strategies for implementing oral health training in primary care practice and safety net settings.[63] Although this is a step in the right direction, logistical challenges remain given that dental and medical systems are so siloed. Telehealth may hold some answers; for example, as many efforts focus on bringing care to where children are. For example, the New York Telehealth Assistants have been successful in bringing oral health screenings, prevention, and referral to inner city schools.[64,65] Receiving preventive services in the primary care setting does not directly translate to obtaining dental care in the future, and physicians are generally dissatisfied with their inability to refer because of a lack of dental providers who will accept their pediatric patients.[46,66,67]

FUTURE RESEARCH

Workforce models to address children's oral health are the focus of current and ongoing research. Although findings are not yet available, these efforts are notable for the scope and level of commitment to understanding impacts on oral health status. In the third round of funding focused on reducing oral health disparities in children, projects funded by the National Institute of Dental and Craniofacial Research (NIDCR) specifically examined workforce policy and new models and their contributions to improving pediatric oral health.[68] A study funded by the Robert Wood Johnson Foundation (RWJF) and being conducted by researchers at the University of California, San Francisco (UCSF) and the University of California, Los Angeles is evaluating 7 workforce innovation models that have the potential to promote prevention and/or achieve improved access to oral health prevention services. Each model will be evaluated for its effectiveness in promoting prevention and its role in contributing to improved oral health outcomes. Projects will also be assessed for fidelity to the original model, their ability to generalize and replicability, and for potential sustainability. RWJF is also funding an evaluation of the Population-centered Risk and Evidence-based Dental Interprofessional Care Team (PREDICT) project, currently underway in Oregon. This quality improvement project is designed to compare traditional practice with a team-based approach of implementing evidence-based guidelines for caries management at the population level. The team includes expanded permit hygienists, community liaisons, dentists and dental specialists, and health IT specialists. Results are expected in late 2017.[69] In addition, the OHWRC, formed as a partnership between the New York Center for Health Workforce Studies and the UCSF, is funded through a 3-year cooperative agreement with the National Center for Health Workforce Analysis of the US Health Resources and Services Administration. A key goal of the OHWRC is to provide timely and accurate data and conduct policy-relevant research to better inform strategies designed to expand access to needed oral health services, particularly for underserved populations. The oral health workforce topic will remain at the top of providers' and policy makers' agendas given how quickly models are changing and developing, the increasing interest in strategies to integrate oral health with primary care, and the critical need for improvement in children's oral health.

DISCUSSION

How does this evidence on the evolving workforce lend itself to delivering better clinical care to children and families? Although undeniably progress has been made in expanding the workforce available to address children's oral health care needs, there is little scholarship on how these changes are affecting clinical care processes, much less individual or population health outcomes. The structural divisions between public health, medical care, and dental care create a challenge not only for care coordination for providers and patients but also for research on the impacts of different models of care.[62]

The policy environment supports some of the innovation now underway, but several significant challenges remain. Expanding pediatric dental coverage through federal and state programs and the ACA has significantly improved oral health access for children in the last decade.[7] Although post-ACA numbers are not yet available, it is likely that use of care by children will continue to increase, and with it the demand for pediatric dental care providers.[70,71] Although this is laudable, a large percentage of the expansion in pediatric coverage is for low-income children and Medicaid programs struggle to attract enough providers, making access for these populations an ongoing problem regardless of workforce sufficiency. States are moving to Medicaid managed care, but the dental field is slow to adopt capitation and lacks the quality and outcome measures, as well as the accountability infrastructure, required to implement value-based payments. A notable exception is Oregon's Coordinated Care Organization program for Medicaid enrollees, in which organizations operate with global budgets and are responsible for all types of health care, including dental care.

For now, the primary strategy being used to achieve cost savings is the use of less expensive labor to provide care wherever safe and effective and to do outreach for education and prevention in community settings. The primary impediment for new models is state-based health professions regulation that requires intense political action for even minor reform and creates artificial barriers to working across professional boundaries.[72]

The dental delivery system is showing signs of rapid transformation toward larger group models and dental service organizations that are actively working to implement evidence-based care practices under evolving financial structures. The pediatric dental care workforce will need to be seamlessly embedded in these models to meet patient needs at a reasonable cost and good value, in organizational settings that are rewarding for providers. The more flexibility these organizations have to design a future workforce and system around patient needs, the more innovative provider teams can be in solving pressing issues for their patients.

SUMMARY

Research examining productivity, quality, and outcomes of traditional pediatric dental care are generally lacking. The literature shows that education, qualifications, and roles are changing with case examples of success, but what these changes portend for patient care remains an open question. New dental team configurations show promise to improve oral health literacy and access to pediatric dental care. However, some workforce innovations are currently geographically restricted to a few areas of the country and often to certain settings or populations. Although shown to be safe and effective within their scope of practice, it is still unclear what impact new dental care providers will have on the care system or population health. In addition, there has been movement in the last decade to engage medical providers in screening, referral, and prevention activities for the oral health care of children, particularly in primary care settings. It is widely acknowledged that improving children's oral health will require a team-based approach. The biggest challenge for the future of pediatric dental care will be how to train, deploy, coordinate, and fund these teams in a patient-centered model of care.

CASE STUDIES

Case study 1: extended care permit registered dental hygienists in Kansas

In 2003, Kansas legislature established the Extended Care Permits for Registered Dental Hygienists (ECP-RDH). There are now 3 levels of ECP-RDHs. An ECP-RDH I can practice in specific settings when a dentist is not present, but with a relationship with a supporting dentist, their own liability insurance, and specific training and practice experience. Services are limited to children receiving specific social services (eg, therapeutic services in nonresidential centers, in foster care, and in public and private schools) who also meet requirements of Medicaid, qualify for free or reduced lunch programs, or other requirements designed to identify children at higher risk for poor access to dental services. ECP-RDH II (added in 2007) can also provide services to persons with developmental disabilities, those 65 years of age and older living in residential care, and those receiving home-based and community-based services. In 2012, a third category was added, ECP-RDH III, which permits the identification of decay and placing an interim dental restoration, adjusting dentures, smoothing a sharp tooth with a low-speed dental handpiece, using local anesthetic (with some limitations), and extracting deciduous teeth (with some limitations). ECP-RDHs must complete a specific course of study and have specified experience as a dental hygienist. The expected clinical care improvement for pediatric oral health is that ECP-RDHs will provide preventive services and some restorative services to high-risk children in underserved settings.

Case study 2: primary dental health aides in Alaska

The Alaska Dental Health Aide (DHA) Program was created in 2005 as a specialty area under the Community Health Aide Program, which has long provided medical services in Alaska's remote communities. There are 4 categories of DHA: primary dental health aides (PDHAs), expanded function dental health aides, dental health aide hygienists, and dental health aide therapists. DHAs focus on prevention, pain relief, infection relief, and basic restorative services. PDHAs practice at 2 levels. The PDHA I level provides dental education and preventive dentistry services, including the application of topical fluorides, after only a few weeks of training in oral hygiene, nutritional counseling, fluoride application, iodine application, and chlorhexidine varnish application. These aides can advance to PDHA II after additional training in at least 1 skill set for this higher level, which can include sealant application, dental prophylaxis, radiographs, and dental assisting. PDHAs practice in both clinics and in remote villages. Within larger communities in which a dental team is present, their work typically focuses on applying fluoride and providing education in both clinic and community settings, such as Head Start programs, nursing homes, and schools. In remote villages, the scope of work is broader, and they are often the sole oral health providers. In the villages, their work often includes examinations of individuals at high risk for caries, including saliva production tests, bacterial load tests, and visual inspection of teeth; application of fluoride varnish in clinic and community settings; instruction in oral hygiene; scheduling of follow-up appointments; and scheduling of appointments when dental teams visit remote communities. The expected clinical care improvement for pediatric oral health is that PDHAs will provide children and families with essential education about oral health, ensure that children receive fluoride treatments, and ensure that those with high caries risk are monitored regularly.

Case study 3: oral health screening and fluoride application in pediatrics offices

Programs to reimburse pediatricians for providing fluoride application to patients often include offering additional training to pediatricians in oral health screening and the development of improved referral processes to pediatric dentists. UnitedHealthcare (UHC) has operated such a program in New Jersey and other states, as part of their medical-dental integrated Medicaid insurance plan. UHC's Chief Dental Officer established close relationships with large pediatrics practices across the state, offering a variety of educational materials about the reimbursement offered, where to order supplies, and local pediatric dentists accepting Medicaid referrals. He also directed pediatricians to training resources, so that they and/or their medical assistants could learn to apply fluoride. UHC's expectation is that this program will both improve the overall health of their pediatric enrollees and reduce long-term costs through effective prevention of dental disease.

Group Health of Puget Sound, an integrated health maintenance organization (now part of Kaiser Permanente), has had a similar program since 2005, for both Medicaid and commercial enrollees. In collaboration with the Washington Dental Services Foundation, they offered in-person training to pediatricians on oral health screening and the application of fluoride varnish. Group Health offered reimbursement to pediatricians for these services, with initial funding from the Foundation. After a successful pilot project, Group Health decided to continue financial support of this program directly and extend it to all clinic sites. The expected clinical care improvement for pediatric oral health is that at-risk children will receive fluoride varnish, more thorough oral health screenings, and more effective referrals to pediatric dentists.

ACKNOWLEDGMENTS

The authors would like to thank Jean Calvo for her research assistance on this article.

REFERENCES

1. US Department of Health and Human Services. Oral health in America: a report of the Surgeon General. Rockville (MD): US Department of Health and Human Services; 2000.
2. US Department of Health and Human Services. National call to action to promote oral health. Rockville (MD): US Department of Health and Human Services, Public Health Service, National Institutes of Health, National Institute of Dental and Craniofacial Research; 2003.
3. Mertz E, Mouradian WE. Addressing children's oral health in the new millennium: trends in the dental workforce. Acad Pediatr 2009;9(6):433–9.
4. Institute of Medicine. The U.S. oral health workforce in the coming decade: a workshop. Washington, DC: The National Academies; 2009.
5. Mertz EA, Finocchio L. Improving oral healthcare delivery systems through workforce innovations: an introduction. J Public Health Dent 2010;70(Suppl 1):S1–5.
6. Nasseh K, Vujicic M. Dental care utilization rate continues to increase among children, holds steady among working-age adults and the elderly. Chicago, IL: American Dental Association; 2015.
7. Nasseh K, Vujicic M. Dental benefits coverage rates increased for children and young adults in 2013. Chicago, IL: American Dental Association; 2015. Available at. http://www.ada.org/~/media/ADA/Science%20and%20Research/HPI/Files/HPIBrief_1015_3.pdf?la=en.
8. Munson B, Vujicic M. Number of practicing dentists per capita in the United States will grow steadily. Chicago, IL: American Dental Association; 2016.

9. Institute of Medicine. Improving access to oral health care for vulnerable and underserved populations. Washington, DC: National Academies Press; 2011.
10. Tsai C, Wides C, Mertz E. Dental workforce capacity and California's expanding pediatric Medicaid population. J Calif Dent Assoc 2014;42(11):757–64, 766.
11. Ramos-Gomez FJ, Silva DR, Law CS, et al. Creating a new generation of pediatric dentists: a paradigm shift in training. J Dent Educ 2014;78(12):1593–603.
12. Massey CS, Raybould TP, Skelton J, et al. Advanced general dentistry program directors' attitudes and behaviors regarding pediatric dental training for residents. J Dent Educ 2008;72(3):344–51.
13. American Dental Association. Surveys of advanced dental education. Chicago: Health Policy Institute; 2015.
14. Santos CL, Douglass JM. Practices and opinions of pediatric and general dentists in Connecticut regarding the age 1 dental visit and dental care for children younger than 3 years old. Pediatr Dent 2008;30(4):348–51.
15. Clark SJ, Duong S, Fontana M. Dental provider attitudes are a barrier to expanded oral health care for children ≤3 years of age. Glob Pediatr Health 2014;1. 2333794X14557029.
16. Long CM, Quinonez RB, Rozier RG, et al. Barriers to pediatricians' adherence to American Academy of Pediatrics oral health referral guidelines: North Carolina general dentists' opinions. Pediatr Dent 2014;36(4):309–15.
17. Salama F, Kebriaei A. Oral care for infants: a survey of Nebraska general dentists. Gen Dent 2010;58(3):182–7.
18. Rutkauskas J, Seale NS, Casamassimo P, et al. Preparedness of entering pediatric dentistry residents: advanced pediatric program directors' and first-year residents' perspectives. J Dent Educ 2015;79(11):1265–71.
19. Casamassimo PS, Seale NS. Adequacy of patient pools to support predoctoral students' achievement of competence in pediatric dentistry in U.S. dental schools. J Dent Educ 2015;79(6):644–52.
20. Seale NS, McWhorter AG, Mouradian WE. Dental education's role in improving children's oral health and access to care. Acad Pediatr 2009;9(6):440–5.
21. Crall JJ, Illum J, Martinez A, et al. An innovative project breaks down barriers to oral health care for vulnerable young children in Los Angeles county. Policy Brief UCLA Cent Health Policy Res 2016;(PB2016–5):1–8.
22. Niederman R, Gould E, Soncini J, et al. A model for extending the reach of the traditional dental practice: the ForsythKids program. J Am Dent Assoc 2008; 139(8):1040–50.
23. Shulman ER, Howard WG, Sharps G, et al. The impact of a continuing education oral health program on providing services for young children by dentists, dental hygienists and dental assistants. J Dent Hyg 2011;85(3):220–8.
24. Solomon ES, Voinea-Griffin AE. Texas first dental home: a snapshot after five years. Tex Dent J 2015;132(6):382–9.
25. Stewart RE, Sanger RG. Pediatric dentistry for the general practitioner: satisfying the need for additional education and training opportunities. J Calif Dent Assoc 2014;42(11):785–9.
26. Delinger J, Gadbury-Amyot CC, Mitchell TV, et al. A qualitative study of extended care permit dental hygienists in Kansas. J Dent Hyg 2014;88(3):160–72.
27. Myers JB, Gadbury-Amyot CC, VanNess C, et al. Perceptions of Kansas Extended Care Permit dental hygienists' impact on dental care. J Dent Hyg 2014;88(6):364–72.
28. Langelier M, Baker B, Continelli T, et al. A dental hygiene professional practice index by state, 2014. Rensselaer (NY): Oral Health Workforce Research Center;

Center for Health Workforce Studies; School of Public Health, SUNY Albany; 2016.

29. Langelier M, Continelli T, Moore J, et al. Expanded scopes of practice for dental hygienists associated with improved oral health outcomes for adults. Health Aff (Millwood) 2016;35(12):2207–15.

30. Post JJ, Stoltenberg JL. Use of restorative procedures by allied dental health professionals in Minnesota. J Am Dent Assoc 2014;145(10):1044–50.

31. Langelier MH, Moore J, Baker B, et al. Case studies of 8 federally qualified health centers: strategies to integrate oral health with primary care. Rensselaer (NY): Center for Health Workforce Studies; School of Public Health, SUNY Albany; 2015.

32. Nash DA. Adding dental therapists to the health care team to improve access to oral health care for children. Acad Pediatr 2009;9(6):446–51.

33. Mathu-Muju KR, Friedman JW, Nash DA. Oral health care for children in countries using dental therapists in public, school-based programs, contrasted with that of the United States, using dentists in a private practice model. Am J Public Health 2013;103(9):e7–13.

34. Pew Charitable Trusts Dental Campaign. States expand the use of dental therapy. Research and Analysis 2016. Available at: http://www.pewtrusts.org/en/research-and-analysis/analysis/2016/09/28/states-expand-the-use-of-dental-therapy. Accessed September 29, 2016.

35. Koppelman J, Vitzthum K, Simon L. Expanding where dental therapists can practice could increase Americans' access to cost-efficient care. Health Aff (Millwood) 2016;35(12):2200–6.

36. Nash DA, Friedman JW, Mathu-Muju K. A review of the global literature on dental therapists. WK Kellogg Foundation; 2012.

37. Bolin KA. Assessment of treatment provided by dental health aide therapists in Alaska: a pilot study. J Am Dent Assoc 2008;139(11):1530–5 [discussion: 1536–9].

38. Urahn SK, Schuler A, Koppelman SG, et al. Expanding the dental team: studies of two private practices. Washington, DC: The Pew Charitable Trusts; 2014.

39. Nash DA, Mathu-Muju KR, Friedman JW. Ensuring access to oral health care for children: school-based care by dental therapists - a commentary. J Sch Health 2015;85(10):659–62.

40. American Dental Association. About community dental health coordinators. Action for Dental Health 2016. Available at: http://www.ada.org/en/public-programs/action-for-dental-health/community-dental-health-coordinators. Accessed September 15, 2016.

41. American Dental Association. Community dental health coordinator. In: Action for Dental Health, editor. Empowering communities through education and prevention. Chicago: American Dental Association; 2016.

42. American Academy of Pediatrics. Oral health risk assessment timing and establishment of the dental home. 2003, 2009. Policy statement. Available at: https://www2.aap.org/oralhealth/PolicyStatements.html. Accessed September 16, 2016.

43. Pahel BT, Rozier RG, Stearns SC, et al. Effectiveness of preventive dental treatments by physicians for young Medicaid enrollees. Pediatrics 2011;127(3):e682–9.

44. Rozier RG, Stearns SC, Pahel BT, et al. How a North Carolina program boosted preventive oral health services for low-income children. Health Aff (Millwood) 2010;29(12):2278–85.

45. Herndon JB, Tomar SL, Catalanotto FA, et al. The effect of Medicaid primary care provider reimbursement on access to early childhood caries preventive services. Health Serv Res 2015;50(1):136–60.

46. Kranz AM, Preisser JS, Rozier RG. Effects of physician-based preventive oral health services on dental caries. Pediatrics 2015;136(1):107–14.

47. Kranz AM, Rozier RG, Preisser JS, et al. Comparing medical and dental providers of oral health services on early dental caries experience. Am J Public Health 2014;104(7):e92–9.

48. Lewis CW, Boulter S, Keels MA, et al. Oral health and pediatricians: results of a national survey. Acad Pediatr 2009;9(6):457–61.

49. Quinonez RB, Kranz AM, Lewis CW, et al. Oral health opinions and practices of pediatricians: updated results from a national survey. Acad Pediatr 2014;14(6): 616–23.

50. Sams LD, Rozier RG, Wilder RS, et al. Adoption and implementation of policies to support preventive dentistry initiatives for physicians: a national survey of Medicaid programs. Am J Public Health 2013;103(8):e83–90.

51. Biordi DL, Heitzer M, Mundy E, et al. Improving access and provision of preventive oral health care for very young, poor, and low-income children through a new interdisciplinary partnership. Am J Public Health 2015;105(Suppl 2):e23–9.

52. Taylor E, Marino D, Thacker S, et al. Expanding oral health preventative services for young children: a successful interprofessional model. J Allied Health 2014; 43(1):e5–9.

53. Kerpen SJ, Burakoff R. Improving access to oral health care for pregnant women. A private practice model. N Y State Dent J 2009;75(6):34–6.

54. Langelier MH, Glicken AD, Surdu S. Adoption of oral health curriculum by physician assistant education programs in 2014. J Physician Assist Educ 2015;26(2): 60–9.

55. Healthcare Performance Consulting. Oral health needs assessment. American Academy of Physician Assistants; March 2013.

56. American Academy of Pediatrics. State Medicaid payment for caries prevention services by non-dental professionals. http://webcache.googleusercontent.com/search? q=cache:9wmh5GcAwEMJ:www2.aap.org/oralhealth/docs/ohreimbursementchart. pdf+&cd=1&hl=en&ct=clnk&gl=us. Accessed March 19, 2017.

57. Langelier M, Surdu S, Gao J, et al. Determinants of Oral Health Screening and Assessment in Physician Assistant Clinical Practice. Rensselaer, NY: Oral Health Workforce Research Center, Center for Health Workforce Studies, School of Public Health, SUNY Albany; December 2016. http://www.oralhealthworkforce.org/wp-content/uploads/2017/03/OHWRC_Oral_Health_Assessment_in_PA_Practice_2016. pdf.

58. Dental providers. 2013. Available at: http://mnchwalliance.org/chws-you/dental-providers/. Accessed September 15, 2016.

59. Healthy Smiles for a Lifetime/Sonrisas Saludables Para Toda La Vida. National Center for Farmworker Health; 2007.

60. [press release]Community health workers are helping Minnesotans access better care. Northwest Technical College; 2016.

61. Quinonez RB, Kranz AM, Long M, et al. Care coordination among pediatricians and dentists: a cross-sectional study of opinions of North Carolina dentists. BMC Oral Health 2014;14:33.

62. Mertz EA. The dental-medical divide. Health Aff (Millwood) 2016;35(12):2168–75.

63. US Department of Health and Human Services. Integration of oral health and primary care practice. Washington, DC: Health Resources and Services Administration; 2014.

64. Kopycka-Kedzierawski DT, Billings RJ. Teledentistry in inner-city child-care centres. J Telemed Telecare 2006;12(4):176–81.

65. Glassman P, Helgeson M, Kattlove J. Using telehealth technologies to improve oral health for vulnerable and underserved populations. J Calif Dent Assoc 2012;40(7):579–85.

66. Miloro B, Vujicic M. Physicians dissatisfied with current referral process to dentists. American Dental Association Health Policy Institute; 2016.

67. Kranz AM, Rozier RG, Preisser JS, et al. Examining continuity of care for Medicaid-enrolled children receiving oral health services in medical offices. Matern Child Health J 2015;19(1):196–203.

68. National Institute of Dental and Craniofacial Research. NIDCR Oral Health Disparities and Inequities Research Consortium. 2015. Available at: http://www.nidcr.nih.gov/research/NIDCR_Centers_and_Research_Networks/Consortium-to-Reduce-Oral-Health-Disparities.htm. Accessed September 7, 2016.

69. Cunha-Cruz J. What is the problem of access to oral care services and improvement in oral health? Cincinnati (OH): National Oral Health Conference; 2015.

70. Yarbrough C, Vujicic M, Nasseh K. More dental benefits options in 2015 health insurance marketplaces. Chicago: American Dental Association; 2015. Available at: http://www.ada.org/~/media/ADA/Science%20and%20Research/HPI/Files/HPIBrief_0215_1.ashx.

71. Meyerhoefer CD, Panovska I, Manski RJ. Projections of dental care use through 2026: preventive care to increase while treatment will decline. Health Aff (Millwood) 2016;35(12):2183–9.

72. Manski RJ, Hoffmann D, Rowthorn V. Increasing access to dental and medical care by allowing greater flexibility in scope of practice. Am J Public Health 2015;105(9):1755–62.

Pediatric Dental-Focused Interprofessional Interventions

Rethinking Early Childhood Oral Health Management

Burton L. Edelstein, DDS, MPH[a,b,*]

KEYWORDS

- Early childhood caries • Social determinants of health • Social workers
- Health educators • Dietitians/nutritionists • Community health workers
- Population oral health • Accountable care/patient-centered medical homes

KEY POINTS

- Early childhood caries (ECC) shares social, environmental, and behavioral determinants with other chronic diseases and conditions that are termed "common risk factors."
- Evidence of effective ECC prevention suggests that prenatal and immediately postnatal interventions work best when delivered by unconventional providers, like helping professionals (eg, social workers, health educators, dietitian/nutritionists) and lay health workers (eg, community health workers).
- Pressures on US health care systems to deliver best outcomes at lowest costs suggest the need for a more efficient and cost-effective approach to early childhood oral health supervision.
- Population-based early childhood health systems hold great potential to allocate resources by risk, improve health care efficiency and cost-effectiveness, and reduce the burden of ECC.
- A tiered delivery system that engages nontraditional providers and serves all young children in a defined population is presented, along with suggestions for research needed for implementation.

Disclosure Statement: I disclose that the early childhood caries research I direct is currently sponsored by the federal Center for Medicare and Medicaid Innovation (C1CMS331347) and report no financial conflicts of interest.

[a] The Columbia University Medical Center, College of Dental Medicine, Section of Population Oral Health, 622 West 168th Street, PH7, Box 20, New York, NY 10032, USA; [b] Children's Dental Health Project, Washington, DC 20036, USA

* The Columbia University Medical Center, 622 West 168th Street, PH17-306, Box 20, New York, NY 10032.

E-mail address: ble22@columbia.edu

THE EARLY CHILDHOOD CARIES PROBLEM

The problem addressed by this contribution is that too many young children suffer from early childhood caries (ECC) that could have been prevented, suppressed, or arrested through adoption of sustained daily salutary behaviors. Too little is known, however, about how to consistently secure those behaviors over time, particularly in high-risk families. This problem is compounded by dentistry's conventional reparative treatment for ECC, which is costly, inefficient, inequitable, and too often fails: a situation that is increasingly untenable in an era of value-based purchasing.

ECC remains highly prevalent and consequential, disproportionately impacting low-income children.[1] Analyses of the 2011 to 2012 National Survey of Children's Health[2] reveal that 10% of poor parents and 7% of working-poor parents report that their young child is not in excellent or very good oral health compared with only 4% of middle-income and 2% of high-income parents. Similarly, poor and working-poor parents report higher levels of dental or oral problems in the past year than do middle-income and high-income parents (16%, 13%, 10%, 6%, respectively). Yet data from Medicaid show that even among poor children, most require little dental care, whereas a small minority ($\sim$5%) account for a high proportion of dental care spending ($\sim$30%).[3]

Like other chronic diseases, caries determinants relate substantially to socially grounded health behaviors rather than clinical factors.[4] Key ECC behavioral determinants are highly cariogenic diets and harmful feeding practices coupled with insufficient exposures to fluorides. Among the relevant social determinants that explain the prevalence of ECC in poor and low-income families are:

- Poverty itself
- Food, income, and housing insecurity
- Low levels of educational attainment and illiteracy
- Lack of social cohesion and discrimination
- Unavailability of healthful foods
- Unfavorable built environments marked by poor-quality housing, crime and violence, and toxic exposures[5]

Healthy People 2020 provides an explanation of how social and environmental risks impact health:

"Health starts in our homes, schools, workplaces, neighborhoods, and communities. We know that taking care of ourselves … influence[s] our health. Our health is also determined in part by access to social and economic opportunities; the resources and supports available in our homes, neighborhoods, and communities; the quality of our schooling; the safety of our workplaces; the cleanliness of our water, food, and air; and the nature of our social interactions and relationships. The conditions in which we live explain in part why some Americans are healthier than others and why Americans more generally are not as healthy as they could be."

Applying this understanding to oral health, Sheiham and Watt[6] recognize that poor diet and hygiene contribute to multiple illnesses and call for an "approach [that] addresses risk factors common to many chronic conditions within the context of the wider socio-environmental milieu," adding that "adopting a collaborative approach is more rational than one that is disease specific." Appreciation of social determinants has also led to calls to "go upstream"[7] when addressing preventable chronic diseases by targeting health behaviors that result in health inequalities.[4] The recognition that social, environmental, behavioral, and epigenetic health determinants are more influential in determining health status than is health care per se[8,9] raises fundamental questions about the limits and limitations of health care and its relationship with educational and support services. In analyzing cross-national differences in health outcomes, Bradley and Taylor[10] note in their 2013 book, *The American Health Care Paradox: Why Spending More Is Getting Us Less*, that other developed countries with better health outcomes not only spend less on health services than does the United States but also spend more on social services that address housing, employment, disability, education, and food security as health determinants.

Nonetheless, there is an important role for clinical care, and the absence of accessible quality dental care contributes to oral health disparities. Unfortunately, despite remarkable improvements in dental care for poor and low-income children,[11] the subpopulations of children at greatest risk for ECC because of nonclinical determinants are also at greatest risk for lack of dental care that is sufficient to meet their needs.[2]

Given the potent forces of social determinants and the ineffectiveness of conventional preventive and therapeutic ECC management (evidence reviewed in the following section), the question at hand is whether conventional dental teams, even in collaboration with conventional medical teams, are best situated to reduce ECC prevalence or whether new interprofessional teams that engage helping professionals and lay health workers may be more effective when assisting at-risk families in the contexts of their lives, homes, and communities.

EVIDENTIARY REVIEW OF CONVENTIONAL FAMILY-LEVEL EARLY CHILDHOOD CARIES BEHAVIORAL INTERVENTIONS

There is little evidence to support conventional educational interventions intended to effectuate sustained daily oral health behavior change.[6,12–14] In their call to integrate oral health with general health promotion, Sheiham and Watt[6] conclude that conventional oral health education is neither effective nor efficient. In a landmark 1996 systematic review and meta-analysis of dental educational interventions, Kay and Locker[12] found that these interventions have "a small positive, but temporary effect on plaque accumulation…; no discernible effect on caries increment, and a consistent positive effect on knowledge levels." A 2013 review largely agreed with these findings, while noting that successful oral health education programs are those that are "labor intensive, involve significant others and have received funding and additional support."[13] Focusing specifically on the effectiveness of oral health education in children, Habbu and Krishnappa[14] also found that clinical improvements are "short-lived" and that knowledge improvements do not lead to proportionate behavioral improvements. A US Preventive Services Task Force (USPSTF) systematic review[15] on prevention of caries in children younger than age 5 found insufficient evidence that screening and counseling by primary care pediatric medical providers reduces ECC experience. A 2013 update to the USPSTF report similarly found a lack of evidence that physician engagement reduces ECC.[16]

The 2016 review by Albino and Tiwari[17] of behavioral research found that motivational interviewing (MI) "represents the most effective [family-level] behavioral strategy to date in terms of caries prevention, as well as changing oral health behaviors." Yet only 1 of 5 supporting studies involved conventional health care providers, physicians, nurses, and administrators in community health centers who were trained by an "experienced nutritionist,"[18] and none involved dentists or dental hygienists. Rather they involved "master's-level therapists,"[19] peer counselors described as "community health representatives" and "local women,"[20] clerical and medical staff at antenatal visits who distributed written materials (reinforced by subsequent mailings),[21] and "dental health educators."[22] Also of note, all studies that reported caries reductions engaged pregnant women[18,20,21] or women who had recently given birth[20,22] rather than parents of dentate children.

Taken together, these findings suggest that conventional health care providers are neither effective nor well positioned in a child's life course to provide effective family-level ECC prevention counseling.

EVIDENTIARY REVIEW OF CONVENTIONAL EARLY CHILDHOOD CARIES DENTAL TREATMENTS

To explore the effectiveness of ECC interventions in young dentate children, the evidence of effectiveness is considered for both medical and surgical approaches.

Medical

Topical chemotherapeutics are available for caries prevention (eg, fluoride varnish, chlorhexidine, xylitol, and povidone iodine) and arrest (silver nitrate, silver diamine fluoride).[23] Preventive agents can be delivered by medical and dental personnel, and arresting agents can be provided by dentists. The USPSTF confirms moderate evidence of effectiveness ("B" level) for fluoride varnish application by medical personnel at the age of tooth eruption. Application of effective agents is also cost-effective relative to repair, as they prevent caries progression in high-risk children at low cost.[24,25] With further study through randomized controlled trials now under way,[26,27] evidence of effectiveness for arresting agents is likely to catch up with pediatric dental educators' enthusiasm for them.[28]

Surgical or Reparative/Restorative Treatments

In sharp distinction to chemotherapeutic approaches, reparative treatments are neither inherently effective nor cost-effective at preventing caries progression. Of necessity, reparative interventions are often provided with the young child under protective stabilization, sedation, or general anesthesia, each of which has recognized benefits and risks[29] and added costs. Dental repair, in the absence of intensive, effective, and sustained behavioral risk-reduction interventions, are short-lived, as dental restorations, with the exception of glass ionomer fillings, are not therapeutic and restorations frequently fail. Among children treated for ECC under general anesthesia, the literature reports caries recurrence rates of 22% to 79%[30–37] at 6 to 36 months after treatment. The youngest children, whose primary dentition is incomplete at the time of repair, are reportedly more likely to demonstrate subsequent caries progression.[37] Restoration failure compounds the problem of caries progression, as Amin and colleagues[38] report that one-third of restored teeth (32.9%) required further treatment over a 3-year follow-up and a significant portion of children, nearly 1 in 10 (8%), require a second dental rehabilitation under general anesthesia. Evidence is largely lacking on which restorative materials are more successful, but amalgam restorations and stainless steel crowns are more often retained.[39,40] When assessed for value, measured as health outcomes per unit cost, these interventions are notably high cost and disappointing in their impact on caries progression.

Yet, extensive repair of primary teeth at a young age is the current standard of care for children with significant ECC. It is supported by professional association policies, current insurance coverage, fee-for-service payment mechanisms, accreditation training requirements in pediatric dentistry, and tradition. It succeeds in eliminating pain and infection, preventing space loss, and improving masticatory function. However, given an understanding of the social and environmental determinants of salutary health behaviors, it is not surprising that caries progression continues even after substantial dental repair.

Cost-effectiveness of early childhood dental care will likely become of ever-greater concern to public and private payers as they seek alternatives that support the "Triple

Aim" of US health care: better health outcomes at lower cost with improved patient experience.[41] Although a thorough review of the cost-effectiveness of current ECC prevention and repair is beyond the scope of this contribution, it is notable that the value propositions for the age-1 dental visit and for dental rehabilitation is questionable because analyses suffer from probable selection bias in both Medicaid[42] and privately insured[43] populations, and available studies engage high-cost dental professional personnel rather than low-cost nonconventional health workers.[44] System dynamics modeling of ECC prevention and management[24,25] finds that all tested interventions reduce caries occurrence and progression but only those that do not involve a health professional are cost saving. Overall, "interventions targeting the highest-risk children provide the greatest return on investment and combined interventions that target ECC at several stages of its natural history have the greatest potential for cavity reduction."[24] In reviewing the limited evidence of effectiveness and cost-effectiveness for early professional dental visits, Lee and colleagues[45] conclude that the rationale for early intervention is strong and that "If appropriate measures are applied sufficiently early, it may be possible to raise a cavity-free child." The question at hand is which health workers are best able to provide caries guidance early enough in a child's life and at a low cost while ensuring a long-term positive outcome.

EVIDENTIARY CONSIDERATION OF NONCONVENTIONAL HEALTH WORKERS

The previously referenced review by Albino and Tiwari[17] of family-level ECC management revealed that all successful programs engaged nondental personnel. Rather, successful programs featured either helping professionals who have engaged in advanced socio-medical training grounded in health behavioral and communications theory and practice or peer counselors who are so alike those they counsel that they have an intuitive understanding of targeted-families' lives. Both are better prepared than dental professionals to address ECC's psychosocial, behavioral, environmental, and cultural determinants. They typically work away from dental facilities in homes and community sites and focus on social and educational predicates of health behaviors as well as those behaviors themselves.

Dental personnel also may serve effectively as helping professionals in ECC counseling,[46,47] but would require sufficient compensation to routinely implement disease management protocols in practice[48] to offset income lost from reductions in dental repair. The high cost of dental professionals and their sophisticated clinical expertise, however, suggest that engaging them in family-level counseling is inherently inefficient while limiting their availability to function at the top of their scope of practice. Improving health care efficiency and effectiveness requires that delegable care be assigned to the least costly competent provider[49] despite the challenges inherent in expanding scopes of practice.[50]

Nonconventional health workers have already been integrated into physical health care to assist patients and their families in disease management and case management. Common to all are their focus on patient-level and family-level engagements, frequent interactions in clinical and nonclinical settings, interest in and ability to directly address social and environmental determinants of health, and capacity to relate to socially disadvantaged families.

Medical Social Workers

Medical social workers (MSWs), long-standing in hospitals with a historical emphasis on case management and discharge planning, are trained to assess social and environmental support needs as patients and their families manage their own health risks and protective factors. MSWs screen and evaluate families' psychosocial and environmental competencies, facilitate understanding of diseases and their management, educate families about the roles of health professionals, facilitate decision making and communication, provide coordinating and navigation services, and arrange for supportive resources.[51] Social work's "multisystem model of case management" also addresses the complexities of adherence to recommended behaviors.[52] As such, social workers are ideally prepared to facilitate families of children with ECC or at risk for ECC to adopt and implement tailored strategies that include goal setting, action planning, and self-management. MSWs have been engaged in dental care, for example, addressing psychosocial barriers to care in Columbia University's student clinics, retaining patients in care at the State University of New York at Buffalo student clinics,[53] and assisting parents whose young children are at risk for ECC at the University of Washington Center for Pediatric Dentistry.[54]

Certified Diabetes Educators

Strong parallels between diabetes and caries control include the need for daily diet management and the analogous management of therapeutics: insulin for diabetes and fluorides for caries. Certified diabetes educators (CDEs) are credentialed diabetes counselors who work in concert with physicians "to promote self-management to achieve individualized behavioral and treatment goals that optimize health outcomes."[55] These counselors, who may be medical professionals, psychologists, pharmacists, occupational therapists, optometrists, podiatrists, dieticians, or social workers,[56] "support informed decision-making, self-care behaviors, problem-solving, and active collaboration with the health care team to improve clinical outcomes, health status, and quality of life,"[57] exactly the components of ECC management needed to prevent, suppress, or arrest its expression. An evaluation by Moran and colleagues[58] concludes that engagement of CDEs "improves clinical outcomes and is cost-effective" and that "diabetes education and support are integral components of diabetes management." More generally, quality-improvement trials based on precepts of chronic disease management have similarly demonstrated effectiveness of such counselors for pediatric diabetes as well as for pediatric asthma.[59] Although CDEs do not typically engage in oral health promotion,[60] their potential roles, responsibilities, training requirements, and deployment in oral health settings have been explored by the American Association of Diabetes Educators.[61] A dentist who elected to train as a CDE advocates for other dentists to pursue this training and more actively engage in clinical management of patients with diabetes.[62]

Certified Health Education Specialists

Like CDEs, certified health education specialists (CHESs) may come from a variety of health-related disciplines, but may also be graduates of bachelor's or higher-level education programs in health, community health, public health, or school health. CHESs must demonstrate competency on examination in 7 defined areas: assessing needs; planning, implementing, evaluating, and administering programs; acting as a resource person; and communicating and advocating.[63] Their work is not disease specific but does address common risk factors for poor health, including poor oral health. No reference to the involvement of CHESs in oral health promotion has yet been identified.

Registered Dietitian Nutritionists

Educated at the bachelor's or higher level, registered dietitian nutritionists (RDNs) complete an accredited curriculum, a supervised internship, and a certifying examination in preparation for individualized diet counseling specific to health conditions and risks, termed medical nutrition therapy. Because ECC has a predominant feeding and diet component, RDNs may be particularly well positioned to assist families in adopting appropriate healthful practices. RDNs assess health histories, eating habits and patterns, and diet content before assisting clients in setting goals and carrying out action plans to reach those individualized goals.[64] The dietetic profession is moving from a "standard educational and informative approach" to "an individualized therapeutic approach" involving "behavioral and lifestyle therapies" that seek to change patients' eating patterns in the context of "cultural needs and desires to achieve sustainable results."[65] Randomized controlled trials and clinical reports validate the effectiveness of RDNs in diabetes management[66] and sustained weight loss and lipid-level improvements.[67] The professional association of RDNs, the Academy of Nutrition and Dietetics, strongly supports integration of oral health with nutrition services, education, and research, noting a "synergistic multidirectional association between diet, nutrition, and oral health."[68] No studies describing the integration of RDNs in dental care were identified.

Community Health Workers

Known by a variety of names, including *promotores*, health navigators, and community health representatives, community health workers (CHWs) are peer counselors who "can improve health access, improve health outcomes, and reduce health care costs for targeted subpopulations."[69] Unlike health professionals and helping professionals who are credentialed and/or licensed, CHWs typically are not and they do not provide clinical services. A 2014 Medicaid regulatory change established a state option under which federally approved state Medicaid plans can allow licensed health care providers (eg, dentists) to delegate preventive services (eg, caries counseling and prevention facilitation) to these nonlicensed health workers. Under this delegation authority, the CHWs are paid directly by Medicaid.[70] A diabetes prevention program offered by the YMCA that has been recognized by the federal Centers for Disease Control and Prevention for its effectiveness and Centers for Medicare and Medicaid Services for its cost-effectiveness engages lay health workers who are called "lifestyle coaches."[71] A dental-specific variant of the CHW is the Community Dental Health Coordinator (CDHCs) advanced by the American Dental Association.[72] Like CHWs, CDHCs engage, educate, and assist at-risk families. They differ, however, in that they are additionally trained to provide a limited set of clinical procedures (eg, coronal polishing and placement of sealants).[73] An ECC intervention with an immigrant Vietnamese population reported that "One-to-one counseling with regular follow-up provided by a lay person of similar background and culture to the participants is an effective way to facilitate adoption of healthy behaviors and to improve oral health of children."[74] Further engagement of CHWs in oral health management has been advocated by the American Academy of Pediatric Dentistry (AAPD) to "enhance provider-patient communication; preventive care; adherence to treatment, follow-up, and referral; disease self-management; and navigation of the health care system." AAPD's policy brief additionally suggests that CHWs can "build individual and community capacity by increasing health knowledge and self-sufficiency through a range of activities, such as outreach, community education, informal counseling, social support, and advocacy among communities such as Hispanic/Latino communities."[75]

Professionals Certified in Public Health

Unique to professionals certified in public health (CPHs) is their focus on improving health of populations rather than individuals by conducting population-level needs assessments and planning, implementing, and evaluating preventive interventions and services that impact groups of people. Although certification is not required of public health professionals, this voluntary credential, validated by examination and continuing education, indicates that "public health professionals have mastered the foundational knowledge and skills relevant to contemporary public health."[76] From a public health perspective, "Strategies to prevent and control ECC should address the dental disease process, promote systems of care that support children during their early developmental years, and develop public health practices for prevention."[77] Common public health approaches important to childhood caries include public education campaigns, population triage efforts to identify highest-risk individuals, community water fluoridation, instituting fluoride varnish programs, and educating health center staff on ECC risks and management.

Further evidence of effectiveness by helping professionals and lay health workers is reported for the federal Home Visiting Program that "gives pregnant women and families, particularly those considered at risk, necessary resources and skills to raise children who are physically, socially, and emotionally healthy and ready to learn."[78] This national program reaches more than 140,000 families of young children whose parents are overwhelmingly poor (77%), with modest education (31% have less than high school education), and are compromised by age (22% are teen parents) and prior experience of abuse (15%) and drug use (12%). Such high-risk families share social determinants with ECC risk. Of the 19 unique programs that have been federally approved to participate in home visiting, "most models had favorable impacts on primary measures of child development and school readiness and positive parenting practices" and 10 of 12 that measured child health improvements demonstrated success.[79] Among the 48 states for which data are available, 10 incorporate dental referral into their Home Visiting Program, 16 provide some level of direct dental service or conduct relevant research, and 22 do not incorporate oral health (unpublished research conducted in 2016 by Sobia Rafiuddin at Columbia University; available from Ms Raffiudin at: sr2782@cumc.columbia.edu).

HOW THIS EVIDENCE CAN BE USED TO DELIVER BETTER CARE TO YOUNG CHILDREN AND THEIR FAMILIES

Taken together, the evidence regarding ECC prevention suggests that the most effective and efficient approaches involve the following:

- Targeting the highest-risk families: those who today receive the least early preventive care
- Starting early, during the perinatal period and well before the first tooth or first birthday
- Involving helping professionals and lay health workers whose training, commitments, and expertise complement that of dental professionals
- Addressing oral health knowledge and enhancing parental capabilities so that families can become active agents for children's overall and oral health
- Tailoring advice and support to the idiosyncratic social, environmental, and cultural conditions in which families live
- Assisting families in accomplishing risk reduction through goal setting, action planning, facilitation, and follow through
- Ensuring the availability of quality dental care for the provision of services that only professional dental personnel can deliver
- Allocating financial and delivery resources proportional to need rather than accepting the current environment in which families self-select for oral health services
- Integrating oral health promotion within programs that address overall health

These principles suggest a new interprofessional population-based model that features 4 cumulative tiers. Each subsequent tier addresses a more narrowly defined group at higher risk for ECC.

Tier 1: Full Population Intervention by Public Health Personnel

The interprofessional model begins by identifying a discrete population of pregnant women and infants. The population may be defined by shared health insurance coverage (eg, those insured by a public or private insurance plan), administration (eg, those enrolled in a managed care plan), service location (eg, those served by a community health center or medical or dental service organization), geography (eg, those in a defined community), program (eg, those enrolled in an Early Head Start Center), health care provider (eg, those under the care of defined obstetricians and pediatricians), or other attribute or combination of attributes that establishes clear inclusion criteria. The entire defined population is served by public health professionals who engage community resources in needs assessment and triage; public education to raise awareness about ECC, its etiologic pathways, risks, and protective factors; and appropriate availability and use of fluorides, including community water fluoridation. Public health personnel additionally work with a range of social services to incorporate ECC prevention within community programs and with Medicaid and Children's Health Insurance Program (CHIP) policymakers to maximize options and opportunities for payment (including, by example, paying CHWs under federal delegation authority).

Tier 2: At-Risk Subgroup Health Promotion and Disease Prevention Interventions by Helping Professionals and Lay Health Workers

The subpopulation of families with elevated risk need to be targeted with more intensive health promotion and disease prevention efforts. Segmentation can be accomplished by using sociodemographic data supplemented with survey or screening findings; by having providers, programs, or insurers identify at-risk families; or by having families self-identify. For example, higher-risk families may be identified as those enrolled in the federal Maternal, Infant, and Early Childhood Home Visiting program; those with a history of intergenerational caries experience or an older child who already experienced ECC; or pregnant women identified by obstetricians, WIC (Women, Infants, and Children) programs, or Early Head Start. Once identified, helping professionals and/or lay health workers will determine, implement, and evaluate strategies to intensify ECC messaging to this population. As with the CPHs in Tier 1, these champions can liaison with a range of social service programs that target families with shared common health determinants to promote inclusion of pediatric oral health.

Tier 3: Acute Risk Group Disease Management Intervention with Helping Professionals and Lay Health Workers

A subset of the Tier 2 population will be those young children at the greatest risk for ECC: those who, if left alone, would be most likely to present with acute symptoms and extensive dental destruction by age 3 years. To meaningfully reduce risk, these families need intensive, personalized, sustained assistance by helping professionals and/or peer counselors who provide individualized education, assistance in goal setting and action planning, and facilitation to accomplish defined goals.

Tier 4: Clinical Dental Intervention

Some families will not respond sufficiently to the proactive interventions detailed in Tiers 1 to 3 and will require corrective dental treatment. In Tier 4, these children are provided care by appropriately trained dentists who deliver both chemotherapeutic and reparative dental services.

The interprofessional population-based oral health approach requires coordination and management across the 4 Tiers. This can be provided by dentists who assume leadership responsibility to develop, implement, and evaluate a system of care designed to meet the needs of all children in the catchment population while integrating with other health promotion programs. Alternatively, coordination and management services may be provided by health systems, particularly emerging accountable care organizations and patient-centered medical homes, or by managed care companies responsible for the group.[80] Financing such a system requires a profound shift from fee-for-service that incentivizes high-volume care to global payment that incentivizes value-based care predicated on objective oral health process or outcome measures. Yet unexplored are methodologies to reward oral health outcomes in early childhood oral health care. At the child level, outcomes may be assessed clinically or by parent reports of their children's oral health status, dental problem, or unmet need for dental care. At the family level, outcomes may be assessed by parent reports of their oral health knowledge and behaviors. At the systems level, outcomes may be assessed by rates of emergency room use for dental complaints and operating room use for dental repair.

The proposed 4-Tier interprofessional population-based model reflects and honors recommended action steps made in 1999 by the Association of Maternal and Child Health Programs[81] and in 2000 by the US Surgeon General's Workshop on Children and Oral Health[82] (**Fig. 1**). The following are the 8 recommendations:

1. "Start early and involve all": This reflects evidence that "early," in the context of ECC prevention, means well before the first tooth or first birthday and even before a child is born. "Involving all" suggests that everyone who can provide authoritative information to families should be engaged to do so within an integrated system of care.
2. "Ensure competencies": This requires that providers of oral health information are competent to do so within the contexts of common risk factors and social determinants of health as well as caries knowledge.
3. "Be accountable": This begs for a care system that measures performance for the entire defined population and allocates resources particularly to those at highest risk.
4. "Take public action": This addresses Tier 1, in which the entire population is addressed to raise awareness and benefit from population-level interventions.
5. "Maximize the utility of science": This calls for retaining fidelity to caries science, behavioral science, communications science, and social science knowledge that is foundational to effective interventions at all Tier levels.
6. "Fix public programs": This suggests that public health and public finance conventions be reconsidered in a movement toward value-based care and incentives inherent to global payments.
7. "Grow an adequate workforce": Today this means a workforce that is competent to serve at each Tier, from public health personnel addressing an entire population to the clinical dentist serving the unique dental treatment needs of an individual child.
8. "Empower families and enhance their capabilities": This acknowledges that ECC risks abide in families and that only successful family engagement can effectively reduce risky behaviors.

An example of a pediatric oral health intervention that reflects many of these principles is the MySmileBuddy (MSB) delivery model that was developed by an interdisciplinary team (pediatric medicine and dentistry, health education, nutrition, social work,

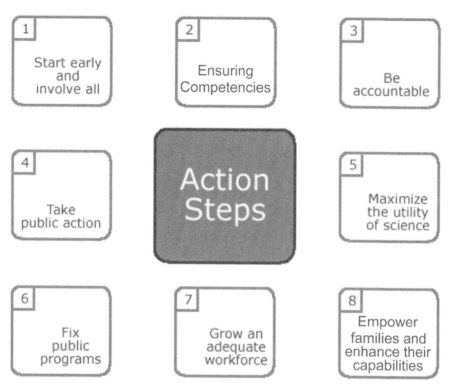

Fig. 1. Action steps to improve young children's oral health. (*From* Columbia Center for New Media Teaching and Learning. Opening the mouth, continuing MCH education in oral health: action steps. Available at: http://ccnmtl.columbia.edu/projects/otm/action.html#one. Accessed September 29, 2016; with permission.)

informatics, and policy) with support from the National Institutes of Health[83] and fielded in an effectiveness trial with support from the federal Center for Medicare and Medicaid Innovation (CMMI).[84] MSB aims to prevent or arrest ECC progression in young at-risk children by pairing their families with technology-assisted CHWs who conduct home visits to educate parents about the determinants and consequences of ECC, assess caries risk, assist parents in establishing family-defined goals and action steps to reduce caries risk and activity, and facilitate accomplishment of those salutary action steps. MSB meets the "start early and involve all" principle by reaching out to families of at-risk children younger than 6 years, developing long-standing family interaction with the CHWs, and linking parents with a range of community housing, food, social, and education services. It "ensures competencies" by empowering families with knowledge, tools (oral hygiene supplies and dietary counseling), and assistance in reaching their self-defined disease management goals. It maximizes the utility of both behavioral and caries science by incorporating key elements of MI and behavioral modification along with dietary counseling and regular toothbrushing with fluoridated toothpastes. As a Medicaid innovation demonstration, MSB seeks to "fix public programs" by demonstrating that nonsurgical caries management in young children is less costly, more effective in obtaining and maintaining oral health, and provides a better patient and family experience than surgical repair of ECC. This intervention contributes to "growing an adequate workforce" by adding

CHWs to the dental team and engaging them in sustained promotion of quotidian oral health behaviors. It "empowers families and enhances their capabilities" by ensuring that they accept control for their children's oral health and act accordingly with as much assistance from the CHW as is appropriate to a given family. Clinical outcomes associated with MSB are pending analysis but narrative reports by CHWs confirm that parents successfully adopt sustained oral health-promoting behaviors.

It is problematic that an interprofessional population-based approach, such as MSB, is at variance with some current professional policies intended to reduce ECC occurrence and progression. The currently recommended universal preventive dental visit by age 1[85–87] in a dental home with a dentist[88] appears from the evidence presented to occur too late to be effective and to be delivered by personnel who are less effective and more costly than nonconventional providers. Logistic constraints on the professionally endorsed early dental home visit[89] additionally tend to favor utilization by low-risk families who are already attuned to oral health, while crowding out or limiting access for families who would benefit most. The proposed model addresses the problem of dealing with parents who are regarded as "not engaged" in their children's oral health,[90] as helping professionals and CHWs are better able to engage parents who may be otherwise overwhelmed by their life circumstances. The proposed model additionally aligns with value-based purchasing changes currently under way in US health care.

FUTURE POSSIBILITIES AND RESEARCH DIRECTIONS TO IMPROVE YOUNG CHILDREN'S ORAL HEALTH

Research is needed to enhance capacity to implement the proposed model by better detailing methods to triage and segment a population by ECC risk, assessing oral health status and care outcomes, providing tiered interventions that are effective and cost-effective, and engaging unconventional health workers in oral health.

Additional experimentation is required to test various insurance designs and payment incentives that can support the tiered interprofessional population-based model, particularly within Medicaid. Future direction can be gained from studying current and past Medicaid policies, including (1) consumer incentives for healthy behaviors,[91] and (2) financing approaches that promote disease management and case management, for example, Primary Care Case Management, the Medicaid Health Home Initiative, State Plan Amendments for Prevention, and Targeted Case Management.

Ongoing unconventional approaches that can inform the interprofessional population-based model include the Iowa I-Smile Program that ensures a dental home for all Medicaid-beneficiary children that does not require a dentist, the Oregon Coordinated Care Organizations that use global payments for oral health services, and the California Medicaid Dental Transformation Initiative that is promoting ECC disease management approaches. The federal CMMI and the National Institute for Dental and Craniofacial Research (NIDCR) also promote unconventional interventions that support a population-based approach. For example, NIDCR underwrote the development of the MSB health information technology[92,93] that CMMI-sponsored CHWs use in home visits to effectuate sustained behavioral change in families whose children already have ECC.[94]

Information relevant to financing of the proposed model will be increasingly forthcoming from experience of nascent accountable care organizations and patient-centered medical homes that are funded by global payments and/or incentivized for positive health outcomes (and financially sanctioned for poor outcomes). Similarly, the increasing occurrence of integrated dental coverage within medical plans, as evidenced in California's and Connecticut's health exchanges, will provide useful experience in promoting financing that cuts across health disciplines.

Overall, application of interprofessional population-based perspectives to the ECC problem holds potential to target children at greatest risk, address their oral health within a larger context of overall health, provide meaningful support for parents who need assistance in providing healthful conditions for their children, improve the family experience with oral health care, and save money. Wrenching as such a novel approach may be to the status quo, it is an evidence-based alternative that synthesizes public health and clinical care for the benefit of all children.

REFERENCES

1. Healthy People 2020 OH-1.1: Children with dental caries in their primary teeth (percent, 3-5 years). Disparities details by income for 2011-12. Available at: https://www.healthypeople.gov/2020/data/disparities/detail/Chart/4992/6.1/2012. Accessed September 23, 2016.
2. Shariff JA, Edelstein BL. Medicaid meets its equal access requirement for dental care but oral health disparities remain. Health Aff (Millwood) 2016;35(12):2259–67.
3. Reforming States Group. Pediatric dental care in CHIP and Medicaid: paying for what kids need, getting value for state payments. New York: Milbank Memorial Fund; 1999. Available at: http://www.milbank.org/uploads/documents/990716mrpd.html. Accessed September 23, 2016.
4. Watt RG. From victim blaming to upstream action: tackling the social determinants of oral health inequalities. Community Dent Oral Epidemiol 2007;35:1–11.
5. Healthy People 2020 Topics and Objectives, Social Determinants of Health. Available at: https://www.healthypeople.gov/2020/topics-objectives/topic/social-determinants-of-health. Accessed September 2, 2016.
6. Sheiham A, Watt RG. The common risk factor approach: a rational basis for promoting oral health. Community Dent Oral Epidemiol 2000;28(6):399–406.
7. Robert Wood Johnson Foundation. BUILD: Going upstraeam to improve community health. 2014. Available at: http://www.rwjf.org/en/culture-of-health/2014/11/build_going_upstrea.html. Accessed September 11, 2016.
8. Centers for Disease Control and Prevention. NCHHSTP social determinants of health. Available at: http://www.cdc.gov/nchhstp/socialdeterminants/faq.html. Accessed September 5, 2016.
9. Health Policy Brief. The relative contribution of multiple determinants to health outcomes. Researchers continue to study the many interconnected factors that affect people's health. Health Affairs. 2014. Available at: http://healthaffairs.org/healthpolicybriefs/brief_pdfs/healthpolicybrief_123.pdf. Accessed September 6, 2016.
10. Bradley EH, Taylor LA. The American Health Care Paradox: why spending more is getting us less. New York, NY: Public Affairs, Perseus Books Group; 2013.
11. Nasseh K, Vujicic M. Dental care utilization rate continues to increase among children, holds steady among working-age adults and the elderly. American Dental Association Health Policy Institute. 2016. Available at: http://www.ada.org/~/media/ADA/Science%20and%20Research/HPI/Files/HPIBrief_1015_1.pdf?la=en. Accessed September 30, 2016.
12. Kay EJ, Locker D. Is dental health education effective? A systematic review of current evidence. Community Dent Oral Epidemiol 1996;24:231–5.
13. Nakre PD, Harikiran AG. Effectiveness of oral health education programs: a systematic review. J Int Soc Prev Community Dent 2013;3(2):103–15.

14. Habbu SG, Krishnappa P. Effectiveness of oral health education in children–a systematic review of current evidence (2005-2011). Int Dent J 2015;65:57–64.

15. US Preventive Services Task Force. Final recommendation statement: dental caries in children from birth through age 5 years: screening. Available at: https://www. uspreventiveservicestaskforce.org/Page/Document/RecommendationStatement Final/dental-caries-in-children-from-birth-through-age-5-years-screening. Accessed September 24, 2016.

16. Chou R, Cantor A, Zakher B, et al. Preventing dental caries in children <5 years: systematic review updating USPSTF recommendation. Pediatrics 2013;132(2): 332–50.

17. Albino J, Tiwari T. Preventing childhood caries: a review of recent behavioral research. J Dent Res 2016;95(1):35–42.

18. Chaffee BW, Feldens CA, Vitolo MR. Cluster-randomized trial of infant nutrition training for caries prevention. J Dent Res 2013;92(7):S29–36.

19. Ismail AI, Ondersma S, Jedele W, et al. Evaluation of a brief tailored motivational intervention to prevent early childhood caries. Community Dent Oral Epidemol 2011;39(5):433–48.

20. Harrison RL, Veronneau J, Leroux B. Effectiveness of maternal counseling in reducing caries in Cree children. J Dent Res 2012;91(11):1032–7.

21. Plutzer K, Spencer AJ, Keirse JM. Reassessment at 6-7 years of age of a randomized controlled trial initiated before birth to prevent early childhood caries. Community Dent Oral Epidemiol 2012;40(2):116–24.

22. Wagner Y, Greiner S, Heinrich-Weltzien R. Evaluation of an oral health promotion program at the time of birth on dental caries in 5-year-old children in Vorarlberg, Austria. Community Dent Oral Epidemiol 2014;42(2):160–9.

23. Milgrom P, Chi DL. Prevention-centered caries management strategies during critical periods in early childhood. J Calif Dent Assoc 2011;39(10):735–41.

24. Hirsch GB, Frosh M, Anselmo T, Edelstein BL. A simulation model for designing effective interventions in early childhood caries. Prev Chronic Dis 2012;9:E66. Epub 2012 Mar 1.

25. Edelstein BL, Hirsch G, Frosh M, et al. Reducing early childhood caries in a Medicaid population: a systems model analysis. J Am Dent Assoc 2015;146: 224–32.

26. Chu CH, Gao SS, Li SK, et al. The effectiveness of the biannual application of silver nitrate solution followed by sodium fluoride varnish in arresting early childhood caries in preschool children: study protocol for a randomised controlled trial. Trials 2015;16:426.

27. Mattos-Silveira J, Floriano I, Fereira FR, et al. New proposal of silver diamine fluoride use in arresting approximal caries: study protocol for a randomized controlled trial. Trials 2014;15:448.

28. Nelson T, Scott JM, Crystal YO, et al. Silver diamine fluoride in pediatric dentistry training programs: survey of graduate program directors. Pediatr Dent 2016; 38(3):212–7.

29. AAPD guideline on behavior guidance for the pediatric dental patient. Pediatr Dent 2015–2016;37(6):180–93.

30. Jamieson WJ, Vargas K. Recall rates and caries experience of patients undergoing general anesthesia for dental treatment. Pediatr Dent 2007;29(3):253–7.

31. Amin MS, Bedard D, Gamble J. Early childhood caries: recurrence after comprehensive dental treatment under general anaesthesia. Eur Arch Paediatr Dent 2010;11(6):269–73.

32. Foster T, Perinpanayagam H, Pfaffenbach A, et al. Recurrence of early childhood caries after comprehensive treatment with general anesthesia and follow-up. J Dent Child (Chic) 2006;73:25–30.
33. Drummond BK, Davidson LE, Williams SM, et al. Outcomes two, three and four years after comprehensive care under general anesthesia. N Z Dent J 2004; 100:32–7.
34. Graves CE, Berkowitz RJ, Proskin HM, et al. Clinical outcomes for early childhood caries: influence of aggressive dental surgery. J Dent Child (Chic) 2004;71(2): 114–7.
35. Eidelman E, Faibis S, Peretz B. A comparison of restorations for children with early childhood caries treated under general anesthesia or conscious sedation. Pediatr Dent 2000;22(1):33–7.
36. Almeida AG, Roseman MM, Sheff M, et al. Future caries susceptibility in children with early childhood caries following treatment under general anesthesia. Pediatr Dent 2000;22:302–6.
37. Amin M, Nouri R, ElSalhyM SP, et al. Caries recurrence after treatment under general anesthaesia for early childhood caries: a retrospective cohort study. Eur Arch Paediatr Dent 2015;16(4):325–31.
38. Amin M, Nouri MR, Hulland S, et al. Success rate of treatments provided for early childhood caries under general anesthesia: a retrospective cohort study. Pediatr Dent 2016;38(4):317–24.
39. Yengopal V, Harneker SY, Patel N, et al. Dental fillings for the treatment of caries in the primary dentition. Chochrane Database Syst Rev 2009;(2):CD004483.
40. Duangthip D, Jiang M, Chu CH, et al. Restorative approaches to treat dentin caries in preschool children: a systematic review. Eur J Paediatr Dent 2016; 17(2):113–21.
41. Institute for Healthcare Improvement. The IHI Triple Aim. Available at: http://www.ihi.org/engage/initiatives/tripleaim/pages/default.aspx. Accessed September 16, 2016.
42. Savage MF, Lee JY, Kotch JB, et al. Early preventive dental visits: effects on subsequent utilization and costs. Pediatrics 2004;114:e418–23.
43. Kolstad C, Zavras A, Yoon RK. Cost-benefit analysis of the age one dental visit for the privately insured. Pediatr Dent 2015;37(4):376–80.
44. Nowak AJ, Casamassimo P, Scott J, et al. Do early dental visits reduce treatment and treatment costs for children? Pediatr Dent 2014;36:489–93.
45. Lee JY, Bouwens TJ, Savage MF, et al. Examining the cost-effectiveness of early dental visits. Pediatr Dent 2006;28:102–5.
46. Ng MW, Torresyap G, White A, et al. Disease management of early childhood caries: results of a pilot quality improvement project. J Heatlh Care Poor Underserved 2012;23(2 Suppl):193–209.
47. DentaQuest Institute. Early Childhood Caries (ECC) Collaborative. Available at: https://www.dentaquestinstitute.org/learn/quality-improvement-initiatives/early-childhood-caries-ecc-collaborative. Accessed September 25, 2016.
48. Ng MW, Ramos-Gomez F, Lieberman M, et al. Disease management of early childhood caries: ECC collaborative project. Int J Dent 2014;2014:327801.
49. Kocher R, Sahni NR. Rethinking health care labor. N Engl J Med 2011;365: 1370–2.
50. LeBuhn R, Swankin DA. Reforming scopes of practice: a white paper. 2010. Citizen Advocacy Center. Available at: https://www.ncsbn.org/Reforming ScopesofPractice-WhitePaper.pdf. Accessed September 25, 2016.

51. National Association of Social Workers Center for Workforce Studies and Social Work Practice. Social workers in hospitals and medical centers: occupational profile. Undated. Available at: http://workforce.socialworkers.org/studies/profiles/Hospitals.pdf. Accessed September 25, 2016.

52. Vourlekis B, Ell K. Best practice case management for improved medical adherence. Soc Work Health Care 2007;44(3):161–77.

53. Zittel-Palamara K, Fabiano JA, Davis EL, et al. Improving patient retention and access to oral health are: the CARES Program. J Dent Educ 2005;69:912–8.

54. University of Washington Pediatric Dental Alumni News. Team Social Work. 2010. Available at: http://thecenterforpediatricdentistry.com/intranet/pednews2010-1.pdf. Accessed July 12, 2016.

55. National Certification Board for Diabetes Educators. What is a CDE? Available at: http://www.ncbde.org/certification_info/what-is-a-cde/. Accessed September 25, 2016.

56. National Certification Board for Diabetes Educators. Discipline requirements. Available at: http://www.ncbde.org/certification_info/discipline-requirement/. Accessed September 25, 2016.

57. National Certification Board for Diabetes Educators. Definition of diabetes self-management education–2016. Available at: http://www.ncbde.org/certification_info/eligibility-requirements/. Accessed September 25, 2016.

58. Moran K, Burson R, Critchett J, et al. Exploring the cost and clinical outcomes of integrating the registered nurse-certified diabetes educator into the patient-centered medical home. Diabetes Educ 2011;37(6):780–93.

59. Edelstein BL, Ng MW. Chronic disease management strategies for early childhood caries: support from the medical and dental literature. Pediatr Dent 2015; 37(3):281–7.

60. Yuen HK, Onicescu G, Hill EG, et al. A survey of oral health education provided by certified diabetes educators. Diabetes Res Clin Pract 2010;88(1):48–55.

61. American Association of Diabetes Educators. AADE thought leader summit: diabetes and oral health. Undated. Available at: https://www.diabeteseducator.org/docs/default-source/default-document-library/aade-diabetes-oral-health-white-paper.pdf?sfvrsn=0. Accessed July 12, 2016.

62. Manchir M. Dentist highlights dentistry's key role in identifying diabetes. American Dental Association News. August 20, 2015. Available at: http://www.ada.org/en/publications/ada-news/2015-archive/august/dentist-highlights-importance-of-dental-role-in-identifying-diabetes. Accessed July 12, 2016.

63. National Commission for Health Education Credentialing, Inc. Available at: www.nchec.org. Accessed September 25, 2016.

64. Academy of Nutrition and Dietetics. What an RDN can do for you. Available at: http://www.eatright.org/resource/food/resources/learn-more-about-rdns/what-an-rdn-can-do-for-you. Accessed September 26, 2016.

65. Endevelt R, Gesser-Edelsburg A. A qualitative study of adherence to nutritional treatment: perspectives of patients and dieticians. Patient Prefer Adherence 2014;8:147–54.

66. Pastors JC, Warshaw H, Daly A, et al. The evidence for the effectiveness of medical nutrition therapy in diabetes management. Diabetes care 2002;25(3):608–13.

67. Welty FK, Nasca MM, Lew NS, et al. Effect of onsite dietitian counseling on weight loss and lipid levels in an outpatient physician office. Am J Cardiol 2007;100:73–5.

68. Academy of Nutrition and Dietetics. Oral health and nutrition. 2014. Available at: http://www.eatrightpro.org/~/media/eatrightpro%20files/practice/position%20 and%20practice%20papers/practice%20papers/practice-paper-oral-health-and-nutrition.ashx. Accessed July 12, 2016.

69. Bovbjerg RR, Eyster L, Ormond BA, Anderson T, Richardson E. The evolution, expansion, and effectiveness of community health workers. 2013. The Urban Institute. Available at: http://www.urban.org/sites/default/files/alfresco/publication-pdfs/413072-The-Evolution-Expansion-and-Effectiveness-of-Community-Health-Workers.PDF. Accessed September 28, 2016.

70. Update on Preventive Services Initiatives. CMCS informational bulletin. 11/27/13. Available at: https://www.medicaid.gov/Federal-Policy-Guidance/Downloads/ CIB-11-27-2013-Prevention.pdf. Accessed September 28, 2016.

71. Centers for Medicare and Medicaid Services. Certification of Medicare diabetes prevention program. March 14, 2016. Available at: https://www.cms.gov/ Research-Statistics-Data-and-Systems/Research/ActuarialStudies/Downloads/ Diabetes-Prevention-Certification-2016-03-14.pdf. Accessed September 28, 2016.

72. American Dental Association. Action for dental health: about community dental health coordinators. Available at: http://www.ada.org/en/public-programs/action-for-dental-health/community-dental-health-coordinators. Accessed September 28, 2016.

73. American Dental Association. Action for dental health: CDHC education and training. Available at: http://www.ada.org/en/public-programs/action-for-dental-health/community-dental-health-coordinators/cdhc-education-and-training. Accessed September 29, 2016.

74. Harrison R, Wong T. An oral health promotion program for an urban minority population of preschool children. Community Dent Oral Epidemiol 2003;31:392–9.

75. Silverman J, Douglass J, Graham L. The use of case management to improve dental health in high risk populations. American Aacdemy of Pediatric Dentistry Oral Health Research and Policy Center. Undated. Available at: http://www. aapd.org/assets/1/7/Case_Management.pdf. Accessed July 12, 2016.

76. National Board of Public Health Examiners. Certified in public health: about NBPHE. Available at: https://www.nbphe.org/aboutNBPHE.cfm. Accessed September 28, 2016.

77. Association of State and Territorial Dental Directors. Early childhood caries policy statement, adopted June 26, 2012. Available at: http://www.astdd.org/docs/early-childhood-caries-policy-statement-june-26-2012.pdf. Accessed September 25, 2016.

78. Health Resources and Services Administration, Maternal and Child Health. Home visiting. Available at: http://mchb.hrsa.gov/maternal-child-health-initiatives/home-visiting. Accessed September 25, 2016.

79. Avellar S, Paulsell D, Sama-Miller E, et al. Home visiting evidence of effectiveness review: executive summary. Washington, DC: Office of Planning, Research and Evaluation, Administration for Children and Families, U.S. Department of Health and Human Services; 2016.

80. Edelstein BL, Rubin MS, Douglass J. Improving children's oral health by crossing the medical-dental divide. Connecticut Health Foundation; 2015. Available at: https://www.cthealth.org/wp-content/uploads/2015/02/Crossing-the-Medical-Dental-Divide-Final.pdf. Accessed September 30, 2016.

81. Association of Maternal and Child Health Programs. Putting teeth in children's oral health policy and programs: the state of children's oral health and the role

of State Title V Programs. 1999. Available at: http://mchoralhealth.org/PDFs/22360.PDF. Accessed September 29, 2016.

82. Edelstein BL. Forward to the background papers from the US Surgeon General's Workshop on Children and Oral Health. Ambul Pediatr 2002;2(2 Suppl):139–40.

83. Chinn CH, Levine J, Matos S, et al. An interprofessional collaborative approach in the development of a caries risk assessment mobile tablet application: my smile buddy. J Health Care Poor Underserved 2013;24:1010–20.

84. The Trustees of Columbia Univerity in the City of New York. MySmileBuddy: Demonstrating the value of technology-assisted non-surgical care management in young children. Available at: https://innovation.cms.gov/initiatives/Health-Care-Innovation-Awards-Round-Two/New-York.html. Accessed January 19, 2017.

85. AAPD guideline on infant oral health care adopted 1986, revised 2014. Pediatr Dent 2015–2016;37(6):146–50.

86. AAPD Guideline on the periodicity of examination, preventive dental services, anticipatory guidance/counseling, and oral treatment for infants, children and adolescents. Pediatr Dent 2015–2016;37(6):123–30.

87. AAPD policy on the dental home adopted 2001, revised 2015. Pediatr Dent 2015–2016;37(6):24–5.

88. AAPD Policy on workforce issues and the delivery of oral health care services in a dental home adopted 2011, revised 2014. Pediatr Dent 2015–2016;37(6):26–31.

89. Edelstein BL. Environmental factors in implementing the dental home for all young children. Rockville (MD): US Department of Health and Human Services, Health Resources and Services Administration, Maternal and Child Health Bureau; 2008. Available at: http://www.usnoha.org/sites/default/files/reports/1.%20Implementing%20the%20Dental%20Home.pdf. Accessed September 30, 2016.

90. AAPD guideline on caries-risk assessment and management for infants and management for infants, children, and adolescents. Pediatr Dent 2016;38(6):142–9.

91. Medicaid and CHIP Payment and Access Commission. Use of healthy behavior incentives in Medicaid. Available at: https://www.macpac.gov/wp-content/uploads/2016/08/The-Use-of-Healthy-Behavior-Incentives-in-Medicaid.pdf. Accessed September 30, 2016.

92. Levine J, Wolf RL, Chinn C, et al. MySmileBuddy: an iPad-based interactive program to assess dietary risk for early childhood caries. J Acad Nutr Diet 2012;112(10):1539–42.

93. Custodio-Lumsen CL, Wolf RL, Contento IR, et al. Validation of an early childhood caries risk assessment tool in a low-income Hispanic population. J Public Health Dent 2016;76(2):136–42.

94. Center for Medicare and Medicaid Innovation. Health Care Innovation Awards Round Two: New York. The Trustees of Columbia University in the City of New York: "MySmileBuddy": demonstrating the value of technology-assisted non-surgical caries management in young children. Available at: https://innovation.cms.gov/initiatives/Health-Care-Innovation-Awards-Round-Two/New-York.html. Accessed September 30, 2016.

Parent Refusal of Topical Fluoride for Their Children

Clinical Strategies and Future Research Priorities to Improve Evidence-Based Pediatric Dental Practice

Donald L. Chi, DDS, PhD

KEYWORDS

- Fluoride refusal • Fluoride hesitancy • Preventive care decision making
- Topical fluoride • Fluoride • Oral health inequalities • Children • Caries risk

KEY POINTS

- Topical fluorides are one of the few evidence-based preventive treatments available and are especially important in preventing dental caries in high-risk children.
- Parent topical fluoride refusal is a growing clinical and public health problem that may contribute to growing pediatric oral health inequalities in the United States.
- The determinants of topical fluoride refusal are complex and multifactorial. Potential solutions include patient-centered social and behavioral interventions that can be easily implemented within clinical settings.
- There are immediate clinical and community-based strategies that can improve parent-provider communication about fluoride and educate the public about the importance of various fluoride modalities.
- Public health researchers need to develop fluoride refusal screening tools, diagnostic instruments, and evidence-based strategies to help parents make optimal preventive dental care decisions for their children.

INTRODUCTION

In the early 1900s, Frederick McKay discovered the oral health benefits of fluoride when he observed that individuals exposed to naturally fluoridated drinking water in Colorado Springs, Colorado were significantly less likely to develop tooth decay.[1] Laboratory studies later confirmed his clinical observations. Since then, topical fluorides have become the cornerstone of prevention in dentistry. Fluoride is available in a variety of modalities each with varying concentrations: drinking water fluoridated

Disclosure Statement: The author has nothing to disclose.
Department of Oral Health Sciences, School of Dentistry, University of Washington, Box 357475, B509 Health Sciences Building, Seattle, WA 98195-7475, USA
E-mail address: dchi@uw.edu

at 0.7 ppm; over-the-counter toothpastes and mouthwashes; foams, gels, and varnishes provided by health providers during dental and medical visits; and prescription-strength toothpastes, drops, or tablets. Fluorides prevent tooth decay by promoting remineralization and inhibiting demineralization of enamel.[2–5] Fluoride is recommended as part of a comprehensive tooth decay prevention program for high-risk children.[6–8] Regular exposure to fluoride is safe, even for young infants.[9,10]

Even though fluoride is effective and safe, recent data showed that 13% of parents refused fluoride treatments for their child during a preventive dental or medical visit.[11] Even more parents are fluoride hesitant, meaning that they may accept fluoride for their children but have unresolved concerns. These are a concern from an evidence-based perspective because fluoride is one of the only preventive treatments available for caries prevention. The growing phenomenon of fluoride refusal has implications for the way in which clinicians communicate with parents about fluoride so that parents can make optimal preventive health care decisions for their children.

This article includes a discussion of conceptual issues related to fluoride refusal, including definitions and measurement-related gaps. Next, the author reviews the relevant scientific literature to identify potential factors related to fluoride refusal. This information forms the basis for recommendations on clinical strategies that can be incorporated into practice and future research priorities related to building on stronger scientific evidence base to manage and address fluoride refusal in clinical settings.

Defining and Conceptualizing Fluoride Refusal

The author defines fluoride refusal as any instance in which a parent has refused, attempted to refuse, or considered refusing professional fluoride therapy for their child in a health care setting because of concerns about the necessity, safety, or consequences of fluoride. The author emphasizes the behavioral, cultural, or social origins of fluoride refusal behaviors rather than developmental or economic causes. Thus, fluoride refusal excludes reasons like a parent refusing because their young child does not like the taste (developmental) or the inability to pay for fluoride treatment when a parent would otherwise accept it (economic).[12,13]

Fluoride refusal is typically conceptualized as a binary behavior. A parent brings their child into clinic, is presented with the option of fluoride, and makes a decision to either accept or refuse fluoride. However, similar to the continuum-of-addiction model used to describe smoking,[14] fluoride refusal is positioned at one end of a continuum that ranges from complete acceptance of fluoride with no reservations to complete refusal with no desire to change one's mind (**Fig. 1**). Somewhere in the middle of this continuum are hesitant parents, regardless of whether they accept fluoride, with some degree of concern. Parents who refuse fluoride are considered hesitant, but not all hesitant parents refuse fluoride. Studies on parent preferences regarding preventive care have reported that most parents accept fluoride, but there are some

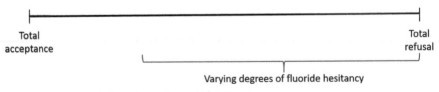

Total
acceptance

Total
refusal

Varying degrees of fluoride hesitancy

Fig. 1. Continuum of fluoride hesitancy behaviors.

parents with concerns.[15,16] These findings support the continuum model. For simplicity, when the author uses the term "fluoride refusal" in this article, it incorporates the concept of hesitancy.

Fluoride Refusal Measurement Gaps

Although broad measures on the acceptability of preventive dental care for children exist,[17] none specifically focus on fluoride. The continuum model indicates the need for 2 types of measures, neither of which currently exist. The first is a screening tool to identify parents who are fluoride hesitant. A screening approach is similar to the process of screening for behavioral health conditions in primary care.[18] Screening tools exist to identify vaccine-hesitant parents. For example, the Parent Attitudes toward Childhood Vaccines is an 18-item measure that addresses beliefs about vaccine safety and efficacy, attitudes, and trust in health providers.[19] The value of a screening tool is that it could help clinicians identify parents who refuse fluoride as well as parents who may accept fluoride for their child but retain some degree of hesitancy. Hesitant parents may be at risk for eventually becoming parents who refuse fluoride. The second is a diagnostic instrument to assess the reason or reasons a parent is hesitant about fluoride. Diagnostic data are critical in developing a logic model of the problem, which describes a problematic health behavior of interest and is a precursor to developing strategies to address the problem behavior based on the underlying reason or reasons for the behavior.[20]

A logic model of the problem, in turn, is needed to develop a logic model of change, which lays out the necessary steps in a causal chain of events that are expected to result in behavior change, in this case reducing fluoride hesitancy and improving fluoride acceptance.[20] There may be a need for multiple logic models because fluoride refusal is a complex, multifactorial health behavior. Multiple logic models form the basis for chair-side interventions tailored to parents based on the specific reason or reasons a parent refuses fluoride.[21]

Reasons for Topical Fluoride Refusal

The origins of fluoride refusal in the United States are traced back to water fluoridation opposition by the John Birch Society during the Soviet era.[22] As such, most relevant studies in the dental literature focus on community resistance to water fluoridation, for which limited knowledge and risk-benefit misperceptions are the main determinants.[23]

There are only 3 publications on topical fluoride refusal. Two publications reported that parents of children with autism spectrum disorders have a higher likelihood of refusing topical fluoride during dental visits.[24,25] Only one other study to date has identified factors related to topical fluoride refusal.[11] In a 3-clinic study in Washington State, fluoride refusal was significantly associated with vaccination refusal.[11] Fluoride refusal was more common among parents under the age of 35 years and those with a college degree.[11] The implication of this study was that a potential strategy to reduce fluoride refusal was to address vaccine refusal. However, subsequent analyses found that different behavioral and social factors were related to vaccination and fluoride refusal behaviors, indicating that different solutions are needed to solve these related problems separately (Carpiano R, Chi DL, unpublished data, 2017).

The association between vaccination and fluoride refusal highlights the relevance of the vaccine literature in identifying the potential causes of fluoride refusal. Similar to topical fluoride, there are more parents who are hesitant about vaccines than those who refuse vaccines.[26] Parent attitudes and beliefs about health are important determinants of vaccine hesitancy. Most common is the belief that vaccines are un-safe and lead to conditions like autism spectrum disorders,[27] which parallel concerns about fluoride. Many parents believe vaccines are no longer necessary.[28–30] These be-liefs are spread through social networks, the media, and anti-vaccine Web sites, where information seeking may be compromised when the parent's primary goals are control and certainty over perceived risks.[31–36] Low health literacy influences the way parents understand and process information about vaccine necessity, safety, and risks.[37] Studies have also found that vaccine refusal is bimodal, with the highest rates present at the highest and lowest ends of the income spectrum, and that the rea-sons for refusal are different for these 2 groups.[38] Other factors include religious be-liefs, a desire for autonomy, and concerns about the true intent of vaccines (ie, financial interest of pharmaceutical companies, government conspiracy).[39–46] These factors have led to a growing number of vaccine-hesitant parents.[19]

Another potential cause of fluoride refusal is rooted within the dental profession and relates to the provision of fluoride treatment that may not always be based on a child's risk for developing caries. A recent Cochrane Review reported caries-prevention ben-efits associated with fluoride varnish in children and adolescents.[5] The studies in this systematic review focused on high-risk children, as is the case with almost all pub-lished fluoride trials. However, not all low-income children are at high risk for caries. This means that recommendations for fluoride should be based on risk, but there is little evidence that this is what actually occurs in practice. Thus, the potential problem is dentists who indiscriminately recommend fluoride varnish for all children regardless of risk. The phenomenon of fluoride refusal in higher-income parents may be a response to recommendations for fluoride treatment when there is little perceived need for fluoride. Fluoride refusal behaviors may also occur in lower-income parents, who may feel disempowered during dental visits because of perceptions that dental offices discriminate against lower-income families.[47] Reactance, a concept from psy-chology that describes parent responses to influences perceived to constrain behav-iors (eg, a dentist telling a parent "all children get fluoride, therefore you should do it"), could help to explain fluoride refusal behaviors.[48]

Fluoride Refusal and Oral Health Inequalities

Although topical fluoride refusal behaviors may occur equally among high- and low-income families, the consequences associated with these behaviors affect the chil-dren differentially. Children from low-income families may be harmed disproportion-ately when they do not receive fluoride because many of these children are at high-caries risk. Children from high-income families who do not receive fluoride oftentimes benefit from other protective factors such as healthier dietary behaviors. Thus, the sociodemographic determinants of fluoride refusal have the potential to lead to increased inequalities between children from higher- and lower-income families. This narrative is consistent with data that fluoride refusal is bimodal—with the highest rates among the lowest- and highest-income families.[11]

Evidence-Based Interventions

Once the epidemiologic factors related to fluoride refusal are identified and the rele-vant logic models are developed, this information can be used to develop tailored chair-side interventions. Although fluoride refusal is multifactorial, it is likely that the reasons can be classified into 4 or 5 typologies, similar to empirical typologies identi-fied in alcohol use and exercise participation.[49,50] Evidence-based intervention ap-proaches can be developed based on each typology to comprehensively address fluoride refusal. For instance, a reactance-based typology might require a behavioral approach that involves shared decision making and consensus building,[51] whereas a fatalism-based typology might focus on emphasizing the possibility of preventing tooth decay and boosting parent self-efficacy to make decisions that increase the odds of disease prevention.[52] Such interventions are developed mainly for parents who refuse fluoride, but can also be delivered to parents exhibiting any degree of fluoride hesitancy. Behavioral informatics–based approaches, which take advantage of technologies and electronic algorithms, could be adopted to deliver precision interventions.[53]

Clinical Strategies

Evidence-based strategies to manage fluoride refusal behaviors in clinical settings have yet to be developed. In the meantime, there are 10 clinical and community-based strategies to help improve communication with parents about topical fluoride and reinforce the importance of fluoride to the public (**Box 1**):

1. *Acknowledge fluoride refusal is a problem.* Some dentists and health professionals may not recognize that there are a significant number of parents concerned about fluoride.[11] These concerns form the basis for fluoride refusal behaviors during preventive health care visits.
2. *Assess parents' knowledge, beliefs, and attitudes about fluoride.* In the absence of validated screening tools that can identify parents who are likely to refuse fluoride, it is important to screen for these behaviors at the start of the preventive visits.[54] Parents should be asked open-ended, nonjudgmental questions[55] that provide an opportunity for starting a conversation about fluoride, like "Fluoride is the sticky stuff dentists paint on children's teeth to prevent cavities. Do you have any questions for me about fluoride?".
3. *Incorporate caries risk into discussions with parents during preventive visits.* Before any recommendations are made about the need for topical fluoride, dentists should explain the child's caries risk to the parent.[56] Anticipatory guidance should be tailored to specific risk factors that manifest in a child and is the starting point to either recommend fluoride (for high-risk children) or explain that fluoride is

---

Box 1
Ten clinical and community-based strategies to help improve topical fluoride-related communication with parents and reinforce the importance of fluoride

1. Acknowledge fluoride refusal is a problem.
2. Assess parents' knowledge, beliefs, and attitudes about fluoride.
3. Incorporate caries risk into discussions with parents during preventive visits.
4. Obtain information about why a parent refuses fluoride.
5. Provide parents a tailored explanation of why topical fluoride is important.
6. If a parent continues to refuse fluoride, discuss alternative fluoride sources and behavioral strategies.
7. Maintain open communication.
8. Accept that some parents will continue to refuse fluoride.
9. Communicate with local health professionals to reinforce the importance of fluoride.
10. Engage in public health advocacy.

not needed at this time (for low-risk children). Low-risk children should not receive fluoride treatment because there is no added health benefit.[57]

4. *Obtain information about why a parent refuses fluoride.* For parents who refuse topical fluoride treatment, pro-fluoride sales pitches should be avoided. Rather, parents should be asked open-ended, respectful questions about the reasons that motivated the parent's decision to opt out of fluoride, like "I respect your decision. Can you tell me some of the reasons that helped you to reach the decision to skip fluoride for your child today?". Listening is a key factor and will help to build trust with a fluoride-hesitant parent.[58] Let the parent speak and avoid interrupting.

5. *Provide parents a tailored explanation of why topical fluoride is important.* It is helpful to provide a tailored explanation of why fluoride is important based on the unique set risk factors associated with each child. For instance, white spot lesions on the child's teeth should be pointed out to the parent, with a description on how fluoride helps to prevent white spots from turning into cavities that require fillings.[59]

6. *If a parent continues to refuse fluoride, discuss alternative fluoride sources and behavioral strategies.* To ensure that high-risk children not receiving professional fluoride are protected from caries, it is important to discuss alternative sources of fluoride that could be used at home, like fluoridated toothpastes and rinsing with fluoride mouthwashes.[8] Twice-daily brushing with fluoride toothpastes should be stressed. Some parents who refuse fluoride during dental and medical visits may be open to use of at-home fluoride products. Other parents avoid all fluoride-containing products. In these latter cases, anticipatory guidance should be framed in the context of the caries balance.[60] If fluorides are not part of the prevention armamentarium, then it is critical for parents to understand that reducing dietary sugars and acids becomes even more critical in managing caries risk.[61,62]

7. *Maintain open communication.* Some parents need to engage in multiple discussions over time before reconsidering their decision to refuse fluoride. Trust is an important aspect of parent decision making. Building trust involves continuity of care, reassurance that the provider respects a parent's health care decisions, and partnership-building communication style.[63] Asking parents for permission to discuss fluoride at future appointments is one way to maintain open communication.[55] It is important to document conversations with parents so that future interactions can be framed appropriately without repeating information and highly sensitive topics can be avoided.

8. *Accept that some parents will continue to refuse fluoride.* Despite repeated attempts at behavior modification, some parents will continue to refuse fluoride. It is important to maintain open communication with parents, monitor the child's caries risk, and incorporate findings from risk assessment into anticipatory guidance. Consistent with professional guidelines from medicine regarding parents who refuse vaccines,[64] fluoride-refusing families should not be dismissed. Some children whose parents refuse fluoride start as high risk but may gradually become low risk (eg, secondary to dietary modification). In these cases, it is important to acknowledge the observed improvements in behavior and the change in caries risk and explain that professional fluorides are not needed as long as healthy behaviors and low-caries risk status are maintained.

9. *Communicate with local health professionals to reinforce the importance of fluoride.* During discussions with parents who refuse fluoride, clinicians may learn about health professionals in the community who are misinforming parents about fluorides.[65] It is helpful to arrange times to meet with these colleagues and discuss the continued importance of fluoride using similar strategies one would use chair

side with fluoride-hesitant parents. Some health providers believe caries rates have reached such low levels that fluorides are no longer necessary. Providing continuing education at medical association meetings can help spread the message that fluorides are important for high-risk children and that all children and adults benefit from lower levels of fluoride found in fluoridated toothpastes and drinking water. The issue of appropriate, risk-based supplementation can also be discussed with professionals who prescribe fluorides to children.[66]

10. *Engage in public health advocacy.* It is also important to educate the public about the importance of fluoride, especially fluoridation of community water supplies. Many individuals are not aware that tooth decay continues to be the most common disease in children and adults. Public advocacy can take place in the form of community outreach events at parent teacher association meetings, editorial pages in newspapers, and education aimed at city council members and state and federal lawmakers.[67]

Research Priorities

There are 4 main research priorities in building the scientific evidence base to address fluoride refusal. First, there is a need for basic epidemiologic research to identify the behavioral, social, and cultural causes of fluoride-refusal behaviors. Second, knowledge about the causes of fluoride refusal should be used to construct fluoride-refusal typologies, each of which will involve a different approach to address fluoride refusal. Testing of these various typology-based approaches in research settings will lead to 4 or 5 approaches that can be combined into a preliminary intervention and tailored to parents based on the specific reasons for fluoride refusal. Third, reliable and valid tools need to be developed that will allow researchers to assess the efficacy of interventions aimed at increasing acceptability of fluoride among parents of high-risk children. These tools can eventually help clinicians identify parents who are likely to refuse fluoride and the reason or reasons for refusal. These tools should be patient-centered (eg, acceptable to patients, nonjudgmental, easy to read and understand) and brief so they can be incorporated into busy clinical settings. Administering these tools electronically could help clinicians with documented and tracking these data in the electronic health record. Fourth, after demonstrating that tailored approaches work in research settings, these programs should be broadly scaled and disseminated into clinical practice.

In conclusion, the growing number of parents who refuse topical fluoride in clinical practice warrants attention from dental professionals and the scientific community. In the short term, there are clinical and community-based strategies available to improve communication with parents about fluoride and educate the public about the importance of fluoride. In the longer term, there is a need to develop measures to identify parents who are likely to refuse topical fluoride and to uncover the reason or reasons for topical fluoride refusal. The goal of this research is to develop evidence-based strategies that can help parents make better preventive dental care decisions for their children, reduce dental disease in high-risk children, and reduce oral health inequalities.

REFERENCES

1. Black GV, McKay FS. Mottled teeth – an endemic developmental imperfection of the teeth heretofore unknown in the literature of dentistry. Dent Cosmos 1916;58: 129–56.

2. Featherstone JD. Prevention and reversal of dental caries: role of low level fluoride. Community Dent Oral Epidemiol 1999;27(1):31–40.

3. Marinho VC, Chong LY, Worthington HV, et al. Fluoride mouthrinses for preventing dental caries in children and adolescents. Cochrane Database Syst Rev 2016;(7):CD002284.

4. Marinho VC, Worthington HV, Walsh T, et al. Fluoride gels for preventing dental caries in children and adolescents. Cochrane Database Syst Rev 2015;(6):CD002280.

5. Marinho VC, Worthington HV, Walsh T, et al. Fluoride varnishes for preventing dental caries in children and adolescents. Cochrane Database Syst Rev 2013;(7):CD002279.

6. Weyant RJ, Tracy SL, Anselmo TT, et al. American Dental Association Council on Scientific Affairs Expert Panel on topical fluoride caries preventive agents. Topical fluoride for caries prevention: executive summary of the updated clinical recommendations and supporting systematic review. J Am Dent Assoc 2013;144(11): 1279–91.

7. Moyer VA, US Preventive Services Task Force. Prevention of dental caries in children from birth through age 5 years: US Preventive Services Task Force recommendation statement. Pediatrics 2014;133(6):1102–11.

8. American Academy of Pediatric Dentistry (AAPD). Guideline on fluoride therapy. Pediatr Dent 2016;38(6):181–4.

9. Milgrom P, Taves DM, Kim AS, et al. Pharmacokinetics of fluoride in toddlers after application of 5% sodium fluoride dental varnish. Pediatrics 2014;134(3):e870–4.

10. Garcia RI, Gregorich SE, Ramos-Gomez F, et al. Absence of fluoride varnish-related adverse events in caries prevention trials in young children, United States. Prev Chronic Dis 2017;14:E17.

11. Chi DL. Caregivers who refuse preventive care for their children: the relationship between immunization and topical fluoride refusal. Am J Public Health 2014; 104(7):1327–33.

12. Humphris GM, Zhou Y. Prediction of nursery school-aged children who refuse fluoride varnish administration in a community setting: a Childsmile investigation. Int J Paediatr Dent 2014;24(4):245–51.

13. Quinonez RB, Kranz AM, Lewis CW, et al. Oral health opinions and practices of pediatricians: updated results from a national survey. Acad Pediatr 2014;14(6): 616–23.

14. Harris JE, Chan SW. The continuum-of-addiction: cigarette smoking in relation to price among Americans aged 15-29. Health Econ 1999;8(1):81–6.

15. Adams SH, Rowe CR, Gansky SA, et al. Caregiver acceptability and preferences for preventive dental treatments for young African-American children. J Public Health Dent 2012;72(3):252–60.

16. Hendaus MA, Jama HA, Siddiqui FJ, et al. Parental preference for fluoride varnish: a new concept in a rapidly developing nation. Patient Prefer Adherence 2016;10:1227–33.

17. Hyde S, Gansky SA, Gonzalez-Vargas MJ, et al. Developing an acceptability assessment of preventive dental treatments. J Public Health Dent 2009;69(1): 18–23.

18. Weitzman CC, Leventhal JM. Screening for behavioral health problems in primary care. Curr Opin Pediatr 2006;18(6):641–8.

19. Opel DJ, Mangione-Smith R, Taylor JA, et al. Development of a survey to identify vaccine-hesitant parents: the parent attitudes about childhood vaccines survey. Hum Vaccin 2011;7(4):419–25.

20. Bartholomew LK, Mullen PD. Five roles for using theory and evidence in the design and testing of behavior change interventions. J Public Health Dent 2011;71(Suppl 1):S20–33.

21. Baker R, Camosso-Stefinovic J, Gillies C, et al. Tailored interventions to overcome identified barriers to change: effects on professional practice and health care outcomes. Cochrane Database Syst Rev 2010;(3):CD005470.

22. McNeil DR. America's longest war: the fight over fluoridation, 1950–. Wilson Q 1985;9(3):140–53.

23. Armfield JM, Akers HF. Community water fluoridation support and opposition in Australia. Community Dent Health 2011;28(1):40–6.

24. Rada RE. Controversial issues in treating the dental patient with autism. J Am Dent Assoc 2010;141(8):947–53.

25. Capozza LE, Bimstein E. Preferences of parents of children with autism spectrum disorders concerning oral health and dental treatment. Pediatr Dent 2012;34(7):480–4.

26. Gust DA, Darling N, Kennedy A, et al. Parents with doubts about vaccines: which vaccines and reasons why. Pediatrics 2008;122(4):718–25.

27. Abu Kuwaik G, Roberts W, Zwaigenbaum L, et al. Immunization uptake in younger siblings of children with autism spectrum disorder. Autism 2014;18(2):148–55.

28. Alfredsson R, Svensson E, Trollfors B, et al. Why do parents hesitate to vaccinate their children against measles, mumps and rubella? Acta Paediatr 2004;93(9):1232–7.

29. Bardenheier B, Yusuf H, Schwartz B, et al. Are parental vaccine safety concerns associated with receipt of measles-mumps-rubella, diphtheria and tetanus toxoids with acellular pertussis, or hepatitis B vaccines by children? Arch Pediatr Adolesc Med 2004;158(6):569–75.

30. Dannetun E, Tegnell A, Hermansson G, et al. Parents' reported reasons for avoiding MMR vaccination. A telephone survey. Scand J Prim Health Care 2005;23(3):149–53.

31. Roberts RJ, Sandifer QD, Evans MR, et al. Reasons for non-uptake of measles, mumps, and rubella catch up immunisation in a measles epidemic and side effects of the vaccine. BMJ 1995;310(6995):1629–32.

32. Calandrillo SP. Vanishing vaccinations: why are so many Americans opting out of vaccinating their children? Univ Mich J Law Reform 2004;37(2):353–440.

33. Fredrickson DD, Davis TC, Arnould CL, et al. Childhood immunization refusal: provider and parent perceptions. Fam Med 2004;36(6):431–9.

34. Lawrence GL, Hull BP, MacIntyre CR, et al. Reasons for incomplete immunisation among Australian children. A national survey of parents. Aust Fam Physician 2004;33(7):568–71.

35. Torun SD, Demir F, Hidiroglu S, et al. Measles vaccination coverage and reasons for non-vaccination. Public Health 2008;122(2):192–4.

36. Gupta VB. Communicating with parents of children with autism about vaccines and complementary and alternative approaches. J Dev Behav Pediatr 2010;31(4):343–5.

37. Smith CA, Ellsworth PC. Patterns of cognitive appraisal in emotion. J Pers Soc Psychol 1985;4(48):813–38.

38. Berezin M, Eads A. Risk is for the rich? Childhood vaccination resistance and a Culture of Health. Soc Sci Med 2016;165:233–45.

39. Slovic P. Perception of risk. Science 1987;236(4799):280–5.

40. Slovic P, Peters E, Finucane ML, et al. Affect, risk, and decision making. Health Psychol 2005;24(4S):S35.

41. Cormick C. Social research into public attitudes towards new technologies. J Verbrauch Lebensm 2014;9(1):3945.

42. Kennedy AM, Gust DA. Measles outbreak associated with a church congregation: a study of immunization attitudes of congregation members. Public Health Rep 2008;123(2):126–34.

43. Grabenstein JD. What the world's religions teach, applied to vaccines and immune globulins. Vaccine 2013;31(16):2011–23.

44. Salmon DA, Omer SB. Individual freedoms versus collective responsibility: immunization decision-making in the face of occasionally competing values. Emerg Themes Epidemiol 2006;3:13.

45. Guidry JP, Carlyle K, Messner M, et al. On pins and needles: how vaccines are portrayed on Pinterest. Vaccine 2015;33(39):5051–6.

46. Tafuri S, Gallone MS, Cappelli MG, et al. Addressing the anti-vaccination movement and the role of HCWs. Vaccine 2014;32(38):4860–5.

47. Lam M, Riedy CA, Milgrom P. Improving access for Medicaid-insured children: focus on front-office personnel. J Am Dent Assoc 1999;130(3):365–73.

48. Brown AR, Finney SJ, France MK. Using the bifactor model to assess the dimensionality of the hong psychological reactance scale. Educ Psychol Meas 2011;71(1):170–85.

49. Norman GJ, Velicer WF. Developing an empirical typology for regular exercise. Prev Med 2003;37(6 Pt 1):635–45.

50. Harrington M, Velicer WF, Ramsey S. Typology of alcohol users based on longitudinal patterns of drinking. Addict Behav 2014;39(3):607–21.

51. Fogarty JS. Reactance theory and patient noncompliance. Soc Sci Med 1997;45(8):1277–88.

52. Finlayson TL, Siefert K, Ismail AI, et al. Reliability and validity of brief measures of oral health-related knowledge, fatalism, and self-efficacy in mothers of African American children. Pediatr Dent 2005;27(5):422–8.

53. Pavel M, Jimison H, Spring B. Behavioral informatics: dynamical models for measuring and assessing behaviors for precision interventions. Conf Proc IEEE Eng Med Biol Soc 2016;2016:190–3.

54. Rose GL, Ferraro TA, Skelly JM, et al. Feasibility of automated pre-screening for lifestyle and behavioral health risk factors in primary care. BMC Fam Pract 2015;16:150.

55. Healy CM, Pickering LK. How to communicate with vaccine-hesitant parents. Pediatrics 2011;127(Suppl 1):S127–33.

56. American Academy of Pediatric Dentistry (AAPD). Guideline on caries-risk assessment and management for infants, children, and adolescents. Pediatr Dent 2016;38(6):142–9.

57. Varsio S, Vehkalahti M. Dentists' decisions on caries risk and preventive treatment by dental state among 15-year-old adolescents. Community Dent Health 1997;14(3):166–70.

58. Holt D, Bouder F, Elemuwa C, et al. The importance of the patient voice in vaccination and vaccine safety-are we listening? Clin Microbiol Infect 2016;22(Suppl 5):S146–53.

59. Guedes RS, Piovesan C, Floriano I, et al. Risk of initial and moderate caries lesions in primary teeth to progress to dentine cavitation: a 2-year cohort study. Int J Paediatr Dent 2016;26(2):116–24.

60. Featherstone JD. Caries prevention and reversal based on the caries balance. Pediatr Dent 2006;28(2):128–32 [discussion: 192–8].
61. Moynihan P, Petersen PE. Diet, nutrition and the prevention of dental diseases. Public Health Nutr 2004;7(1A):201–26.
62. Marshall TA. Preventing dental caries associated with sugar-sweetened beverages. J Am Dent Assoc 2013;144(10):1148–52.
63. Horn IB, Mitchell SJ, Wang J, et al. African-American parents' trust in their child's primary care provider. Acad Pediatr 2012;12(5):399–404.
64. Diekema DS, American Academy of Pediatrics Committee on Bioethics. Responding to parental refusals of immunization of children. Pediatrics 2005; 115(5):1428–31.
65. Weatherspoon DJ, Horowitz AM, Kleinman DV. Maryland physicians' knowledge, opinions, and practices related to dental caries etiology and prevention in children. Pediatr Dent 2016;38(1):61–7.
66. Sohn W, Ismail AI, Taichman LS. Caries risk-based fluoride supplementation for children. Pediatr Dent 2007;29(1):23–31.
67. Galer-Unti RA, Tappe MK, Lachenmayr S. Advocacy 101: getting started in health education advocacy. Health Promot Pract 2004;5(3):280–8.

Precision Dentistry in Early Childhood

The Central Role of Genomics

Kimon Divaris, DDS, PhD[a,b,]*

KEYWORDS

- Children • Oral health • Dentistry • Precision medicine • Genomics

KEY POINTS

- Genomics' role is now well characterized for rare and penetrant developmental traits of early childhood, including craniofacial malformations and developmental defects of dental hard tissues.
- Children have demonstrably varying individual susceptibilities to dental caries; however, specific loci, genes, and implicated pathways, functions, and environmental interactions remain elusive.
- Dental caries is etiologically heterogeneous but mostly behaviorally driven—half of its observed variance may be attributable to predisposing genomic factors that interact with common, modifiable risk factors.
- Genomics likely influences early childhood caries (ECC) susceptibility via control of dental anatomy, enamel quality, salivary properties, immunity, oral microbiome composition, taste preference, and other intermediate characteristics.

EARLY CHILDHOOD CARIES AND PRECISION HEALTH CARE

During the last few there have been remarkable improvements in understanding of the underpinnings of children's oral health, including the fundamental proximal and distal determinants of oral diseases. Translating this body of evidence to actionable knowledge has not been realized to its full potential, and coordinated interdisciplinary efforts are warranted.[1] The elimination of oral health disparities should arguably be the first priority in any research and policy agenda.[2] A parallel and synergistic goal remains

Disclosure Statement: The author has nothing to disclose.
Funding Source: The study was funded by the National Institute of Dental and Craniofacial Research of the National Institutes of Health (grant U01DE025046).
[a] Department of Pediatric Dentistry, UNC School of Dentistry, University of North Carolina at Chapel Hill, 228 Brauer Hall, CB#7450, Chapel Hill, NC 27599, USA; [b] Department of Epidemiology, Gillings School of Global Public Health, University of North Carolina at Chapel Hill, 2101 McGavran-Greenberg Hall, CB #7435, Chapel Hill, NC 27599, USA
* Department of Pediatric Dentistry, UNC School of Dentistry, 228 Brauer Hall, CB#7450, Chapel Hill, NC 27599.
E-mail address: Kimon_Divaris@unc.edu

the development of optimal, personalized oral health care, tailored to individual profiles, risk factors, and innate susceptibilities—a notion termed, *precision dentistry*.[3,4]

Precision dentistry is aligned with the precision medicine initiative—a contemporary approach in health care that takes into account individual differences due to people's genetic makeups, environments, and lifestyles. Initially, precision medicine was introduced in the context of cancer treatment but its longer-term aim is to inform health care, including health promotion as well as prevention and treatment of chronic disease.[5] Although the concept is not fundamentally new (eg, blood typing is a simple yet long-established practice), it has the potential to bring about catalytic changes in health care if informed by recent advances in genomics and other omics applications. The demands for more and better data to support these initiatives are higher than ever, with the need for million-participant cohorts[6] and deep phenotyping[7] frequently articulated. Such biologically informed data from population-based cohorts are still scant in the oral health domain, with few recent examples in periodontal research.[8,9] Early molecular evidence exists, however, to support individual differences to caries susceptibility and fluoride exposure[10] and predisposition to dental fear and anxiety,[11] both of which could inform the customized oral health care (eg, periodic recall frequency and preventive care plans).

In the pediatric oral health domain, ECC persists as the most common chronic childhood disease with substantial human, economic, and societal impacts.[12] The disease disproportionately affects minorities and socioeconomically disadvantaged families, who also face barriers of access to care. The problem of high disease burden combined with inadequate opportunities for prevention and treatment, referred to as a twin disparity,[13] has substantial social and economic implications and has a direct impact on children's oral health outcomes as well as the quality of their health care. It is unsurprising that despite decreases in the disease prevalence among other age groups, ECC rates have remained high. The overwhelming influence of social determinants of health is an undeniable reason for this trend.[2] With that important backdrop, other possible explanations for the persistence of this early-onset, aggressive form of childhood dental caries must look beyond established behavioral, environmental, and societal risk factors and consider biological ones.

THE HERITABILITY OF EARLY CHILDHOOD CARIES AND GENETIC STUDIES TO DATE

The notion of a genetic basis of oral traits and dental diseases, including dental caries, is not new. Early evidence from twin studies[14,15] supports the heritability of dental caries, whereas more recent estimates of heritable variance in childhood caries explained by genetics are in the range of 40% to 70%[16–19]; and this susceptibility seems independent of sweetness preference heritability.[20] Despite an understanding of the importance of genomics for ECC, knowledge of specific ECC risk-conferring polymorphisms is limited. Initial results from candidate gene studies have highlighted genes involved in amelogenesis, immunity, and sweet taste preference[21–23]; nevertheless, none of these early findings has been validated and replicated as a robust, risk polymorphism for dental caries or ECC, specifically. This is not surprising given the small sample sizes of most studies to date, the fact that candidate-gene results tend to show very low replication rates in subsequent genome-wide scans, and other common research design limitations.[24,25]

RECENT GENOME-WIDE ASSOCIATION EVIDENCE

Genome-wide association studies (GWAS) offer an improvement over conventional candidate-gene studies—they entail the simultaneous interrogation (ie, association testing with a trait of interest) of millions of single nucleotide polymorphisms (variable areas of the genome) without being limited to specific areas of the genome due to prior hypotheses.[26,27] GWAS are not meant to provide answers regarding causal evidence or mechanistic explanations in complex diseases but can highlight areas of the genome (ie, loci) that offer promising candidates for further experimentation. The first-ever GWAS of primary dentition caries (children ages 3–12) discovered suggestive evidence of association for 7 genetic loci,[28] 2 of which (MPPED2 and ACTN2) were replicated in a subsequent investigation.[29] Additional key findings from this new line of research using the GWAS methodology are that genetic influences on dental caries may differ between the primary and the permanent dentition[30] as well as between tooth surfaces (ie, smooth vs pits and fissures).[19] Although these results require further validation and replication, they may reflect different biological pathways in play, different interaction patterns with environmental exposures like fluoride and diet, or other unknown or unmeasured factors. In sum, this line of research so far underscores the importance of considering the intraoral heterogeneity of dental caries susceptibility in the context of precision dentistry.[3]

It must be acknowledged that these early findings have been generated from nonminority populations (ie, mainly of European descent) whereas only few children under the age of 6 (the upper age limit for ECC) have been included in the analytical samples. Although validated and replicated loci and genetic pathways for ECC remain largely elusive, the knowledge base of oral health genomics in early childhood is rapidly expanding and holds substantial promise. As the evidence base on the genomics of ECC widens, it is foreseeable that risk loci (ie, gene polymorphisms, regulatory areas, or other functional elements of the human genome) will be discovered and validated as contributors to ECC—given the multifactorial nature and high prevalence of the disease, it may be anticipated that a large number of loci each contribute to a small degrees to ECC resistance of development, according to the paradigm of Manolio and colleagues.[26] The introduction and consideration of more biologically informed endophenotypes and biological proximates[3,31] of ECC (eg, microbial plaque metabolome and transcriptome, salivary proteome) in the GWAS context will help further elucidate the molecular basis of the disease pathogenesis, a necessary piece of the precision dentistry puzzle.

GENETIC REGULATION OF INTERMEDIATE CHARACTERISTICS—ENDOPHENOTYPES

Genetic influences may be hard to identify when considering multifactorial clinical dental endpoints (eg, a decayed, missing due to caries and restored tooth surfaces index) that are affected by upstream factors, including access to dental care. The key regulatory role of the genome on oral and dental traits, however, may be possibly discerned with higher fidelity when considering more proximal, biological endpoints, often called endophenotypes. Such promising targets include dental anatomy, enamel quality, salivary properties, immunity, oral microbiome composition, and others.[3] From a mechanistic standpoint, the regulation of dental tissue (eg, enamel, dentin, cementum, and pulp) formation may be a first-target domain for the study of genetic contributions on both physiologic development and pathology. Accordingly, substantial progress has been made on the genetics front of ectodermal dysplasias and associated dental manifestations, including aberrations in tooth number (eg, hypodontia and oligodontia), size, and shape.[32–34]

GENOMIC CONTROL OF ODONTOGENESIS

A recent investigation by Hu and colleagues[35] found that thousands of genes are implicated in amelogenesis and dentinogenesis, with a subset of genes differentially expressed between these 2 developmental processes. Importantly, enamel is the dental tissue that is first affected by dental caries and it may be expected that developmental defects of the enamel predispose to ECC.[36] Wright and colleagues[37] offer an excellent review of genes and processes involved in enamel formation, including cell differentiation; production and processing of extracellular matrix; altering of cell function during different stages of enamel formation; cell movement and attachment; regulation of ion and protein movement; regulation of hydration, pH, and other conditions of the microenvironment; and more. Unraveling the complexity and diversity of molecular pathways involved in tooth development is certainly a key for the next steps in personalized, precise dental care—including bioengineering, regenerative dentistry applications,[38] and even the prospect of dental rehabilitation via whole-tooth regeneration.[39]

THE GENOMIC BASIS OF OTHER ORAL HEALTH TRAITS

A model example of another, genetically controlled condition with important oral health implications is the family of orofacial clefts—these birth defects comprise congenital malformations of the oral cavity and the face. The environmental and genetic underpinning of orofacial clefts has been the focus of major collaborative research efforts.[40] Although a comprehensive characterization of the genetic basis of various subtypes of orofacial clefts has yet to be accomplished, substantial progress has been made in the discovery of implicated genetic loci in diverse ancestral populations, as recently reviewed and reported by Dixon and colleagues.[41] Other conditions include ectodermal dysplasias[42,43] and other issues related to histodifferentiation, apposition, and mineralization, including amelogenesis imperfecta, dentinogenesis imperfecta, and dentin dysplasia—all these conditions have profound impacts on the oral health functioning and related quality of life of affected individuals and require specialized, precise oral health care.[42]

NECESSARY STEPS TO ADVANCE THE SCIENCE AND PRACTICE OF EARLY CHILDHOOD ORAL HEALTH CARE

The need for a solid evidence base to advance the science and practice of dentistry is undeniable.[43,44] Above and beyond more and better data at all levels (from genes to communities), other features are equally important for an agenda that advances and promotes oral health in childhood—these include but are not limited to interdisciplinary collaboration to maximize synergies and population impact; understanding the full spectrum of individual, cultural, and societal factors having an impact on oral health and related behaviors; engaging and ultimately empowering communities to take control and create healthy environments; and advocating for wellness-promoting and socially responsible policies at all levels.[13,45,46]

A VISION FOR PRECISION DENTISTRY IN PEDIATRIC ORAL HEALTH CARE

Advancements in the science underlying pediatric oral health care will be based on a thorough understanding of the biology of oral health and disease, including the key orchestrating roles of the genome and the oral microbiome as well as the science of behavior change, nutrition (specifically sugar-related policies), and technological innovation. The introduction of biosensors is certain to revolutionize oral health self-monitoring at home or remotely, similar to stem cell research transforming dental rehabilitation options. The promotion of precision dentistry, however, should not be done at the expense of efforts aimed at reducing and ultimately eliminating health disparities via upstream action—at first, it may seem that the 2 approaches are to some degree antagonistic when research funding decisions or inferences regarding individuals need to be made.[47] In the long run, the translation of precise oral health care into socially responsible practices, interventions, and policies can bring about the desired equitable and sustainable population-level oral health improvements.

REFERENCES

1. Casamassimo PS, Lee JY, Marazita ML, et al. Improving children's oral health: an interdisciplinary research framework. J Dent Res 2014;93(10):938–42.
2. Lee JY, Divaris K. The ethical imperative of addressing oral health disparities: a unifying framework. J Dent Res 2014;93(3):224–30.
3. Divaris K. Predicting dental caries outcomes in children: a "risky" concept. J Dent Res 2016;95(3):248–54.
4. Kusiak JW, Somerman M. Data science at the National Institute of Dental and Craniofacial Research: changing dental practice. J Am Dent Assoc 2016; 147(8):597–9.
5. Collins FS, Varmus H. A new initiative on precision medicine. N Engl J Med 2015; 372(9):793–5.
6. Sankar PL, Parker LS. The precision medicine initiative's all of us research program: an agenda for research on its ethical, legal, and social issues. Genet Med 2016. http://dx.doi.org/10.1038/gim.2016.183.
7. Delude CM. Deep phenotyping: the details of disease. Nature 2015;527(7576): S14–5.
8. Offenbacher S, Divaris K, Barros SP, et al. Genome-wide association study of biologically informed periodontal complex traits offers novel insights into the genetic basis of periodontal disease. Hum Mol Genet 2016;25(10):2113–29.
9. Morelli T, Moss KL, Beck J, et al. Derivation and validation of the periodontal and tooth profile classification system for patient stratification. J Periodontol 2017; 88(2):153–65.
10. Shaffer JR, Carlson JC, Stanley BO, et al. Effects of enamel matrix genes on dental caries are moderated by fluoride exposures. Hum Genet 2015;134(2): 159–67.
11. Randall CL, Shaffer JR, McNeil DW, et al. Toward a genetic understanding of dental fear: evidence of heritability. Community Dent Oral Epidemiol 2016. http://dx.doi.org/10.1111/cdoe.12261.
12. Casamassimo PS, Thikkurissy S, Edelstein BL, et al. Beyond the dmft: the human and economic cost of early childhood caries. J Am Dent Assoc 2009;140(6): 650–7.
13. Edelstein BL. Dental care considerations for young children. Spec Care Dentist 2002;22(3 Suppl):11S–25S.
14. Goodman HO, Luke JE, Rosen S, et al. Heritability in dental caries, certain oral microflora and salivary components. Am J Hum Genet 1959;11:263–73.
15. Horowitz SL, Osborne RH, Degeorge FV. Caries experience in twins. Science 1958;128:300–1.
16. Dawson DV. Genetic factors appear to contribute substantially to dental caries susceptibility, and may also independently mediate sucrose sweetness preference. J Evid Based Dent Pract 2008;8:37–9.
17. Ballantine JL, Zandona AF, Zeldin LP, et al. Genome-wide association study of early childhood caries: a pilot study. J Dent Res 2016;94(Spec Iss A):2411969.

18. Shuler CF. Inherited risks for susceptibility to dental caries. J Dent Educ 2001;65: 1038–45.
19. Shaffer JR, Wang X, Desensi RS, et al. Genetic susceptibility to dental caries on pit and fissure and smooth surfaces. Caries Res 2012;46(1):38–46.
20. Bretz WA, Corby PM, Melo MR, et al. Heritability estimates for dental caries and sucrose sweetness preference. Arch Oral Biol 2006;51:1156–60.
21. Shimizu T, Ho B, Deeley K, et al. Enamel formation genes influence enamel micro-hardness before and after cariogenic challenge. PLoS One 2012;7:e45022.
22. Kulkarni GV, Chng T, Eny KM, et al. Association of GLUT2 and TAS1R2 genotypes with risk for dental caries. Caries Res 2013;47:219–25.
23. Briseño-Ruiz J, Shimizu T, Deeley K, et al. Role of TRAV locus in low caries expe-rience. Hum Genet 2013;132:1015–25.
24. Tabor HK, Risch NJ, Myers RM. Candidate-gene approaches for studying com-plex genetic traits: practical considerations. Nat Rev Genet 2002;3(5):391–7.
25. Ioannidis JP, Ntzani EE, Trikalinos TA, et al. Replication validity of genetic associ-ation studies. Nat Genet 2001;29(3):306–9.
26. Manolio TA, Collins FS, Cox NJ, et al. Finding the missing heritability of complex diseases. Nature 2009;461(7265):747–53.
27. Visscher PM, Brown MA, McCarthy MI, et al. Five years of GWAS discovery. Am J Hum Genet 2012;90(1):7–24.
28. Shaffer JR, Wang X, Feingold E, et al. Genome-wide association scan for child-hood caries implicates novel genes. J Dent Res 2011;90:1457–62.
29. Stanley BO, Feingold E, Cooper M, et al. Genetic Association of MPPED2 and ACTN2 with Dental Caries. J Dent Res 2014;93:626–32.
30. Wang X, Shaffer JR, Weyant RJ, et al. Genes and their effects on dental caries may differ between primary and permanent dentitions. Caries Res 2010;44(3): 277–84.
31. Nyvad B, Crielaard W, Mira A, et al. Dental caries from a molecular microbiolog-ical perspective. Caries Res 2013;47(2):89–102.
32. Bergendal B, Norderyd J, Zhou X, et al. Abnormal primary and permanent den-titions with ectodermal symptoms predict WNT10A deficiency. BMC Med Genet 2016;17(1):88.
33. Bergendal B. Orodental manifestations in ectodermal dysplasia-a review. Am J Med Genet A 2014;164A(10):2465–71.
34. Bergendal B, Klar J, Stecksén-Blicks C, et al. Isolated oligodontia associated with mutations in EDARADD, AXIN2, MSX1, and PAX9 genes. Am J Med Genet A 2011;155A(7):1616–22.
35. Hu S, Parker J, Wright JT. Towards unraveling the human tooth transcriptome: the dentome. PLoS One 2015;10(4):e0124801.
36. Caufield PW, Li Y, Bromage TG. Hypoplasia-associated severe early childhood caries–a proposed definition. J Dent Res 2012;91(6):544–50.
37. Wright JT, Carrion IA, Morris C. The molecular basis of hereditary enamel defects in humans. J Dent Res 2015;94(1):52–61.
38. Amrollahi P, Shah B, Seifi A, et al. Recent advancements in regenerative dentistry: a review. Mater Sci Eng C Mater Biol Appl 2016;69:1383–90.
39. Oshima M, Tsuji T. Whole tooth regeneration as a future dental treatment. Adv Exp Med Biol 2015;881:255–69.
40. Gowans LJ, Adeyemo WL, Eshete M, et al. Association studies and direct DNA sequencing implicate genetic susceptibility loci in the etiology of nonsyndromic orofacial clefts in sub-Saharan African populations. J Dent Res 2016;95(11): 1245–56.

41. Dixon MJ, Marazita ML, Beaty TH, et al. Cleft lip and palate: understanding genetic and environmental influences. Nat Rev Genet 2011;12(3):167–78.

42. Innes NP, Evans DJ, Clarkson JE, et al. Obtaining an evidence-base for clinical dentistry through clinical trials. Prim Dent Care 2005;12(3):91–6.

43. American Academy of Pediatric Dentistry. Guideline on dental management of heritable dental developmental anomalies. Pediatr Dent 2013;35(5):E179–84.

44. AAPD's evidence-based dentistry initiative. Available at: http://www.pediatric dentistrytoday.org/2013/September/XLIX/5/news/article/281/. Accessed March 17, 2017.

45. Edelstein BL. Public and clinical policy considerations in maximizing children's oral health. Pediatr Clin North Am 2000;47(5):1177–89, vii.

46. Watt RG. From victim blaming to upstream action: tackling the social determinants of oral health inequalities. Community Dent Oral Epidemiol 2007;35(1): 1–11.

47. Khoury MJ, Galea S. Will precision medicine improve population health? JAMA 2016;316(13):1357–8.

Research Evidence Use in Early and Periodic Screening, Diagnostic, and Treatment Dental Medicaid Class Action Lawsuits

CrossMark

Stephanie Cruz, MA*, Donald L. Chi, DDS, PhD

KEYWORDS

- Medicaid • Research evidence • Policy decision making • Research use • EPSDT
- Dental services • Evidence-based dentistry • Children

KEY POINTS

- Dentists had key roles in 2 cases that required scientific expertise or clinical experience based on an understanding of vulnerable populations.
- Most research evidence in the 2 cases was newly generated data rather than based on existing data.
- The conceptual model linking actors to research evidence helps to further delineate the role of dentists in Medicaid lawsuits and indicates that dentists were involved in all phases of the lawsuit.
- The study underscores individual and collective social justice as the ultimate goals of dental Medicaid lawsuits against states brought forth by marginalized populations and raises the question of the degree to which justice was actually served.

INTRODUCTION

The Early and Periodic Screening, Diagnostic, and Treatment (EPSDT) program was enacted in 1967 to ensure that Medicaid-enrolled children have access to health care services, including comprehensive dental care. Nevertheless, access to dental care has been limited for many children in Medicaid. The barriers to care are well-documented.[1-7] To address this problem, Medicaid enrollees have filed lawsuits against state Medicaid programs alleging EPSDT violations, resulting in consent decrees, which are settlements that enforce the provision of EPSDT dental benefits

Disclosure Statement: The authors have no disclosures.
Department of Oral Health Sciences, School of Dentistry, University of Washington, Box 357475, B509 Health Sciences Building, Seattle, WA 98195-7475, USA
* Corresponding author.
E-mail address: stefcruz@uw.edu

Dent Clin N Am 61 (2017) 627–644
http://dx.doi.org/10.1016/j.cden.2017.03.001
dental.theclinics.com

to child Medicaid enrollees.[8] Two recent EPSDT lawsuits resulted in consent decrees: *Frew v Ladd* and *Hawkins v Commissioner*.

Frew v Ladd (Civil No. 3:93CV65) was initiated in 1993 in Texas (**Table 1**). There were 4 claims against the state:

1. Failure to inform families about EPSDT dental benefits
2. Underperformance on annual dental utilization goals, with only 17% of eligible children receiving a dental screening
3. Failure to provide follow-up treatment after screenings
4. Differential provision of dental services to Medicaid-enrolled versus privately insured children.

In 1995, after 2 years of evidence collection, negotiations, and drafting of the consent decree, a federal court in Texas ruled that the class had standing. The consent decree was deemed to be fair and enforceable. After the *Frew* court determined that the state was violating the consent decree, the state appealed to have the consent decree terminated. In 2004, the US Supreme Court ruled that the consent decree did not violate the constitution and agreed with the district court ruling to uphold the consent decree. Some of the remedies within the consent decree have been implemented. The case is ongoing.

Hawkins v Commissioner (Civil No. 99–143-JD) was filed in 1999 in New Hampshire (see **Table 1**). In 2004, a New Hampshire federal court ruled that the class had standing. The negotiated consent decree was deemed fair and enforceable. The *Hawkins* consent decree was enforced for 5 years. It ended in 2010 after a 1-year extension when the court determined the state had met the terms of the consent decree.

Dental lawsuits provide opportunities to understand how research evidence is used and generated. Both cases relied on research evidence at various stages, but the extent to which research evidence was used is unclear. This is a concern from an evidence-based perspective because these processes may not always take into account available scientific evidence.[9] Knowledge exchange frameworks have been used to conceptualize interactions between researchers, policymakers, and practitioners.[10] These frameworks identify actors and the interactions between actors and research evidence.[11–14] Previous work in dentistry has examined the connections between research, policy, and health care reform, but no studies to date have used knowledge exchange frameworks to understand the use of research evidence in dental Medicaid lawsuits.[15–18]

The goal of the study was to better understand how research evidence is part of legal and policymaking processes in dental Medicaid lawsuits. Based on case studies from Texas and New Hampshire, there were 3 study aims:

1. To identify the main actors in dental lawsuits
2. To characterize the research evidence either used or generated
3. To develop a conceptual model describing the relationship between actors and research evidence.

METHODS

This was a 2-phase qualitative study involving archival analyses and key informant interviews. We used archived documents from each case to identify the case dockets and focused on the claims and findings of fact in the original complaints, transcripts of the court hearing, court decisions, and consent decrees.[19,20] Legal documents were obtained from the Public Access to Court Electronic Records (PACER) service.[21] For the archival analyses, we focused on 8 case dockets (**Table 2**).

Table 1
Procedural timeline of *Frew* and *Hawkins* lawsuits

Linda Frew, on behalf of her daughter, Carla Frew, et al, v Richard Ladd, Commissioner of the Texas Health and Human Services (HHS) Commission, et al	Cassandra Hawkins et al, v Commissioner, New Hampshire (NH) Department of HHS (DHHS)

Eastern District of Texas Court

Year	Procedural Action	Holdings
1993	Complaint filed	Lawsuit filed on behalf of the class of Medicaid-enrolled children in Texas
1995	Fairness hearing	2-day hearing on the lawsuit and proposed settlement
1996	Consent decree approved	Court found the class had standing and the consent decree fair and enforceable
1998	Motion to enforce consent decree	Plaintiffs argued that the state had not carried out parts of the consent decree and asked the court to enforce the settlement
2000	Memorandum of opinion	Judge held that defendants violated parts of the consent decree and that the decree was enforceable

New Hampshire District Court

Year	Procedural Action	Holdings
1999	Complaint filed	Lawsuit filed on behalf of the class of Medicaid-enrolled children in New Hampshire
2003	Consent decree hearing	Court heard arguments over the proposed settlement
2004	Consent decree and order approving consent decree and motion to enforce settlement approved	Court found the class had standing and the consent decree fair and enforceable
2006	Court-appointed mediator	Plaintiffs and defendants were in dispute over whether the NH DHHS was complying with the consent decree The court appointed a mediator to address the dispute Mediation was unsuccessful
2007	Order denying motion to enforce consent decree	Plaintiffs filed motion to enforce the consent decree Court ordered plaintiffs to file supplemental motion clarifying relief sought and put the NH DHHS

(continued on next page)

Table 1
(continued)

Year	Event	Year	Outcome
			on notice that grounds may exist to support contempt
2003	5th Circuit Court of Appeals reverses consent decree enforcement ruling	2008	Order denying motion for contempt and for further relief	Court ruled that the consent decree is in violation of 11th Amendment	Court concluded plaintiffs had not met the standard showing that the NH DHHS should be held in contempt for failing to comply with the consent decree
2004	US Supreme Court reverses 5th Circuit Court of Appeals decision	2010	Order denying motion for contempt and motion to modify consent decree	Court found the consent decree was enforceable	Court again concluded plaintiffs did not show why NH DHHS should be held in contempt and denied motion to extend consent decree for 3 y
2007	Corrective action order signed	—	—	Court enforced original consent decree plus 11 modifications put forth by defendants	—
2013	Memorandum of opinion	—	—	Some corrective action orders from 2007 were satisfied but remaining orders and the consent decree remained in effect	—
2017	Case is ongoing	—	—	—	—

Shaded area indicates period of analysis for study.

Table 2
Case docket documents for *Frew* and *Hawkins* lawsuits used in archival analyses

Case	Year Filed	Document Number[21]	Description
Frew	1993	1	Original complaint
	1995	197	Transcript of fairness hearing before judge
	1996	133	Order concerning fairness of consent decree
	1996	135	Consent decree
Hawkins	1999	1	Original complaint
	2003	1456	Transcript of proceedings for consent decree hearing
	2004	213	Order approving motion to enforce settlement, and granting motion to approve consent decree
	2004	214	Consent decree

Based on the archival analyses, we developed a semistructured script for the key informant interviews (**Box 1**). Discussion topics included:

1. Interviewee's role in the case and connections to other actors
2. Perceptions on barriers and facilitators of dental care for Medicaid children
3. The use or generation of research evidence in the lawsuit
4. Consent decree remedies.

Case dockets were used to identify potential study participants who were recruited by phone or email. We used purposive and snowball sampling techniques to identify additional participants.[22] We interviewed 6 attorneys, 3 expert consultants, 1 expert witness, 3 practitioner witnesses, and 2 state health administrators. To ensure anonymity, we excluded additional information about the interviewees.

Participants consented verbally. Interviews were conducted by phone, lasted 60 to 90 minutes, and were digitally recorded. The recordings were transcribed by a

Box 1
Semistructured script for key informants' interviews

Description of the interviewee's involvement
How did you become involved in the case?
What was your relationship to the issue?

Description of dental access for Medicaid-enrolled children
What was the state of dental care access for Medicaid children before the lawsuit was filed?
What part of this triggered the lawsuit?
Was there disagreement over this?
What were some of the proposed measures before filing the lawsuit?
Who proposed them? What kind of data did they use as evidence? How were they negotiated?

Description of the use of research evidence
Who were the key players in the lawsuit? How did they participate? What kind of expertise did they contribute?
What influence did literature (academic journal articles, agency generated white papers, news articles) have as evidence?

Description of the consent decree remedies
Tell me about the process that led to increased reimbursement rates for dentists.
Tell me about the process to update the registry or lists of dentists.
Tell me more about the process of doing outreach and education for dentists and patients.

professional transcription service. The accuracy of each transcript was verified before analysis.

We used a knowledge exchange framework to guide data analyses.[10,14,23] Data were coded inductively to identify the actors, describe the types of evidence used or generated, and to delineate the relationships among the actors and evidence. We used a content analysis approach to analyze the data and develop a conceptual model.[24] The study was approved by the Institutional Review Board of the University of Washington.

RESULTS
Question 1. Who Were the Actors in the Dental Medicaid Lawsuits?

There were 5 categories of actors: beneficiaries, attorneys, evidence purveyors, judges, and implementers (**Table 3**).

Beneficiaries
These were Medicaid-enrolled children who failed to receive dental care (referred to as plaintiffs). Beneficiaries initiated the lawsuits with the help of legal aid lawyers. As 1 dentist explained

> Pretty much everything [legal aid] do[es] is motivated by [beneficiaries] coming to them seeking legal help. [Legal aid] didn't start by saying, "We're going to take on a cause." It is more that they have been working trying to help individual clients and they were hearing this repeated over and over again–that [dental care access] was a problem.

A legal aid attorney explained they "had a lot [of clients] that had dental problems with real small children...their teeth were rotting out and these parents didn't know that they could even get treatment or where."

Attorneys
Responsibilities of plaintiff and defense attorneys included deposing witnesses, preparing information for review by opposing counsel, requesting and collecting research evidence, negotiating the consent decree, and prioritizing remedies.

Plaintiff attorneys Plaintiff attorneys pursued legal action on behalf of beneficiaries. The main goal was to prove the state had violated EPSDT by failing to provide dental care to children. Once the case moved forward, plaintiff attorneys drafted the initial consent decree remedies and negotiated the final consent decree with defense attorneys.

Defense attorneys According to a defense attorney, the state "maintained it was complying with Medicaid and EPSDT requirements for dental care." The initial goal was to get the case dismissed by attributing low utilization rates to dentists who refused to treat Medicaid patients and families that failed to obtain care for their children. After the consent decree was deemed enforceable, defense attorneys were then responsible for demonstrating improvements to the Medicaid dental program so the consent decree would be dismissed.

Evidence purveyors
These actors produced data, provided testimony, and interpreted research for the attorneys. The actors were state health administrators, practitioner witnesses, expert witnesses, and expert consultants.

State health administrators State health administrators provided attorneys with raw claims and eligibility data from the Medicaid program and dental utilization information

Table 3
Descriptions and roles of actors in *Frew* and *Hawkins* lawsuits

Actor	Description	Role
Beneficiaries	Medicaid-enrolled children and families in Texas and New Hampshire, referred to as plaintiffs or the class	Initiated lawsuits, provided affidavits, depositions, and testimony on their experiences navigating Medicaid services
Attorneys		
Plaintiff Attorneys	Legal aid organizations in Texas and New Hampshire who represented the plaintiffs	Deposed witnesses, prepared information for review by opposing counsel, requested and collected research evidence, negotiated the consent decrees, and prioritized remedies
Defense Attorneys	Texas and New Hampshire Attorney General offices or the state's legal counsel in HHS	
Evidence Purveyors		
State Health Administrators	State health administrators including state Medicaid Directors and dental Medicaid Directors	Supplied attorneys with research evidence on state dental Medicaid programs by sharing dental utilization rates, surveying practitioners, providing recommendations on dental screening schedules, or using expertise in dental research
Practitioner Witnesses	Dentists and state dental association representatives	
Expert Witnesses	Local academic researchers affiliated with public health programs and dental schools	
Expert Consultants	Nationally recognized academic and legal health researchers	
Judges	Federal judges who arbitrated the class action lawsuits in the Eastern District of Texas and New Hampshire District Courts	Listened to the evidence presented in support of the consent decree, evaluated the remedies, arbitrated on the appropriateness and fairness of the consent decree, enforced the consent decree, and could hold the state in contempt if it failed to carry out terms of the consent decree
Implementers		
State HHS Commissioner	The Commissioner of the Texas HHS Commission or NH DHHS, referred to as the defendant	Implemented the consent decree remedies to broaden access for and treat Medicaid-enrolled children
Practitioners	Dentists who would ultimately be responsible for providing care to children in Medicaid	

generated for the Centers for Medicare and Medicaid Services (CMS). These actors included the state Medicaid Director and dental Medicaid Director.

Administrators for the defense explained how policies before the lawsuit were based on outdated professional standards. For example, parents were told that a child's first dental visit should occur by age 3 years and not by age 1 year as recommended by the American Academy of Pediatric Dentistry. A state health administrator explained "there weren't dental or health people running" the Medicaid program. Another example was the American Dental Association guideline recommending 2 preventive dental visits each year as a metric for tracking dental utilization for children.

When they used this metric, they found that dental utilization rates for the state "were abysmal." An administrator explained that the consent decree had prompted the state Medicaid program to consult with professional organizations and experts within dental schools to ensure that assessment measures were based on up-to-date professional standards.

Practitioner witnesses Practitioner witnesses shared their experiences providing care to Medicaid-enrolled children and representing the profession's interests. These actors included dentists and state dental association representatives.

In both states, practitioner witnesses agreed that dental care access was a problem for children in Medicaid. A plaintiff attorney explained that "some of the dentists who started refusing to participate in the Medicaid dental program…would tell us that it just wasn't affordable." In addition, dentists mentioned "paperwork hassles" as the other major barrier to Medicaid participation. The paperwork was complex and Medicaid program staff was not always available to answer questions. Another issue was "swamping" when an overwhelming number of patients would seek care from the only Medicaid dentist in a local area. State dental association representatives presented data on the number of practicing dentists in the state as well as clinical guidelines.

Expert witnesses Expert witnesses testified on various aspects of the consent decree, including remedies to solve the problems with Medicaid. Expert witnesses included local academics affiliated with public health programs and dental schools. Unlike practitioner witnesses, expert witnesses provided data-based rather than anecdotal testimonies. A plaintiff attorney said that selecting expert witnesses did not mean telling the witness "'here is exactly what we want you to say.'…We sent them copies of the [consent decree]…then we asked them what they thought about particular things…They would tell us and we would follow up with more probing questions."

Expert witness testimonies helped attorneys craft evidence-based remedies, such as coverage of dental sealants in children who might not otherwise receive them. Policies to reimburse dentists for sealants on Medicaid-enrollees older than age 14 years in the *Frew* consent decree were based on expert witness testimony on "the [varying] eruption patterns of children and teeth, [meaning] not every child would be able to have this done by the 14th birthday…the lifting of that age limit widen[ed] the window [to] provide this preventive procedure."

Expert consultants These actors provided attorneys with data to set the context for legal arguments and develop consent decree remedies but did not testify in court. Expert consultants included nationally recognized academic researchers. One plaintiff attorney explained that expert consultants "helped frame the complaint…not only writing the complaint, but what kinds of [dental] issues were most important and how those issues in general related to our clients' particular experience." Other responsibilities included "advising us about what kinds of provisions would be the most helpful in settlement negotiations and also what [the expert witness] thought about the provisions the state was proposing and why they might not work" and how to implement consent decree remedies. An expert consultant explained that his role was to "interpret what was going on… [and provide] an independent analysis of [the state's] data."

Judges
Judges directly influenced the policy making process based on their ability to approve or deny the consent decree. The judges in *Frew* and *Hawkins* did not draft the consent

decree but had the plaintiff and defense attorneys work together to negotiate a document. Judges listened to the evidence presented in support of the consent decree, evaluated the proposed remedies, and arbitrated on the appropriateness and fairness of the consent decree. Judges eventually approved consent decrees in both states. Afterward, their primary responsibility was to enforce the terms of the consent decree. Judges could hold a state in contempt or order other remedies if the state failed to carry out agreed on terms.

Implementers

These actors were responsible for implementing the remedies, either by enacting policies to encourage dentists to treat children in Medicaid or providing dental care services. There were 2 types: the state Health and Human Services (HHS) commissioner and practitioners.

State Health and Human Services commissioner The state HHS commissioner was the defendant named in the lawsuits but "once the judge ordered him to do something, the state HHS commissioner became the implementer." The commissioner was responsible for requesting additional funding from the state legislature to finance remedy implementation, for appointing directors to administer the Medicaid program, and for overseeing programs aimed at eliminating barriers to care (eg, transportation, insufficient beneficiary knowledge about benefits, shortage of Medicaid dentists). One attorney described the state HHS commissioner as "very astute politically...this guy was adept at moving the money to where the lawsuits were...[he] moved money to the Medicaid dental program to hire more staff" that enabled the state to carry out the consent decree remedies.

Practitioners Practitioners were the dentists who would ultimately be responsible for providing care to children in Medicaid. These dentists worked in private practice offices, community health centers, and dental management organizations. When reimbursement rates were increased as part of the consent decree remedies, more dentists were expected to become active Medicaid providers. Dentists and their supporting staffs received administrative training on how to process Medicaid claims to minimize delays and rejections. Practitioners also received "cultural sensitivity training" consisting of "modules...about the realities of EPSDT recipients' lives to attempt to improve providers' attitudes toward recipients," including limited access to telephone services to schedule and cancel appointments, transportation difficulties, and a lack of childcare.

Question 2: What Research Evidence Was Generated and Used in the Lawsuit Process?

Research evidence was presented through depositions, affidavits, expert consultations, and witness testimonies. There were 2 types of research evidence. The first was use of existing evidence and the second was generation of new evidence.

Use of existing research evidence

In the *Frew* case, dental utilization rates were initially derived from the annual 416 reports the state was required to submit to CMS. These 416 reports contained basic information about EPSDT, such as the number of children who received dental screenings, treatment referrals, and follow-up treatment. These reports were used to monitor individual state performance and allow for state and national comparisons.

Attorneys used federal reports and academic journal articles to document the barriers to dental care for low-income children. Based on the research literature, witnesses provided testimonies on ways to improve oral health. One witness explained sealants "are the most effective preventive technology since fluoride" but noted that many dentists in clinical practice were not placing sealants. Published research was used to justify remedies. An attorney recalled:

An article was published [comparing] the cost of early preventive dental care...to the cost of treating dental problems in kids who didn't get early preventive dental care...cost is always a consideration for the state...the primary focus is on the health of the children and the well-being of the children, but if you have research that shows that something is cost-effective, then that helps both sides.

Generation of new research evidence
The *Hawkins* consent decree involved generating dental utilization rates that were empirically derived from claims data provided by the Medicaid program. Baseline and multiple follow-up analyses were conducted by expert consultants to monitor progress on consent decree remedies.

In *Frew*, the oral health status of Medicaid-enrolled children was evaluated via clinical assessment to estimate the percentage of children with dental disease and the numbers of children requiring hospitalization for treatment of dental disease. Initially, plaintiff and defense attorneys implemented a 1-time clinical assessment. Disputes arose regarding the specific number and quality of subsequent assessments that would be completed. Nevertheless, as the case progressed, contention arose:

Because some of the things plaintiffs wanted us to look at [as health outcomes] were things that we couldn't do from claims data alone. They really wanted [multiple assessments of] health outcomes, but when you're stuck with only administrative data, there's really a lot of limits to what you could do about health status. They wanted...quality of life inventories...and it was just prohibitively expensive...But we ultimately agreed to a set of... [claims-based] measures.

Defense and plaintiff attorneys also commissioned new research to help substantiate legal arguments based on local data. Lawyers worked with state dental associations to administer surveys to dentists as a way to identify the reasons for low participation in Medicaid. An expert consultant found that "dentists weren't that busy and they could see these patients." Two of the main barriers to dental care were low reimbursement rates and the perception of bad beneficiary behavior, such as being more likely to miss appointments as well as the perception that Medicaid patients do not follow health care instructions.

Texas state health administrators collected qualitative research from beneficiaries to measure client satisfaction that they "couldn't address with the claims administrative data" alone. In addition, defendants in *Frew* commissioned a focus group with beneficiaries in Texas that was cited by the judge as "confirm[ing] many problems that plaintiffs allege." For instance, focus group data corroborated the claim "that the attitudes of [dentists] and [dentists'] staff are discouraging to the patients" because dentists did not understand the patients' life difficulties, prompting many patients to skip subsequent dental appointments.

Question 3: What Were the Relationships Between Actors and Research Evidence?
Our conceptual model delineates the relationship between actors and how research evidence was generated and used in the Medicaid dental litigation process (**Fig. 1**).

Frew and *Hawkins* began when beneficiaries contacted plaintiff attorneys because they were unable to obtain dental care (see **Fig. 1**A). Plaintiff attorneys gathered the beneficiaries' grievances over the course of multiple years before filing suit against

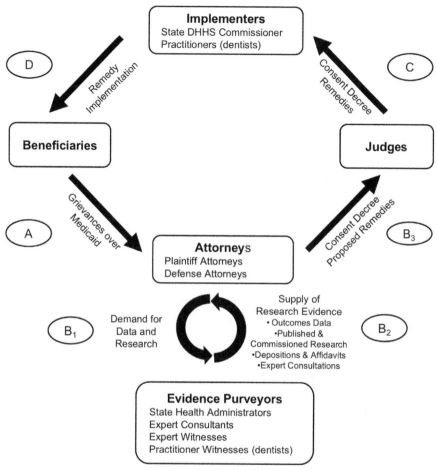

Fig. 1. Relationship between actors and research evidence in *Frew* and *Hawkins* lawsuits (A–D).

the defendants. A plaintiff attorney described this process as "noticing trends. You start noticing people coming in with problems. 'I can't see a dentist', especially in these rural areas. [Or] 'I can't find a dentist that will take Medicaid, so I can't get my child's dental checkups.'"

After the lawsuits were filed, plaintiff attorneys went to state health administrators to obtain dental utilization data. Plaintiff and defense attorneys argued over the state Medicaid program's ability to produce "data on Medicaid dental care because they had archived it and…it would cost them a ton of money to resurrect the data from the storage space to someplace that we, [the plaintiffs], could actually read it or use it." An expert consultant with *Hawkins* noted the difficulties obtaining data because the state "didn't really understand the difference between asking for a report as opposed to asking for a copy of the data." The court eventually ruled that the state had to produce the data at their own expense.

Once Medicaid data were obtained, attorneys asked expert consultants to analyze the data and generate utilization rates (see **Fig. 1B$_1$**). Attorneys also requested data on dentists' experiences with Medicaid as well as other sources of research such as outcomes data, reports, and peer-reviewed publications (see **Fig. 1B$_2$**). Additionally, attorneys from both sides collected affidavits and depositions from state health administrators and witnesses to craft their arguments about the effectiveness or ineffectiveness of the state's Medicaid program. One plaintiff attorney said their expert witness provided "information about the medical aspect of the dental care...she was providing [us] with a lot of research on [tooth decay]... [She] was a pediatric dentist so she was very knowledgeable about...[the] research being done."

With ongoing input from expert witnesses and consultants, plaintiff and defense attorneys worked together to write and negotiate the final consent decree (see **Fig. 1B$_3$**). According to 1 of the attorneys, "we met every day for weeks on end." One practitioner witness recalled the process involved "lots of negotiations back and forth on how is the best way to make known [which dentists accept] Medicaid" because relying on counts of dentists who at 1 point accepted Medicaid was an inaccurate way to compile a registry. He explained that "in New Hampshire there are 600 dentists [on record] that see Medicaid and they are all over the state. That is not the case...in reality, maybe there are 75 that actually see a number of Medicaid kids."

The negotiations in both cases were contentious at times but relations improved over time with both sides focusing on "do[ing] what we need to do for the kids" and eventually coming together to address the problems everyone acknowledged. According to an expert consultant, this was a unique aspect of the consent decree negotiation and writing process because before the lawsuits:

> There [were] standard of care issues. The state's bureaucrats don't know. They are not dental people. They don't know what the standard of care should be or what the services are that should be available and they make rules, arbitrary rules, and sometimes it happens that they get advisory committees made up of people who are not scholarly, who don't know the literature.

Once the proposed remedies were registered in court, the judges called a hearing to listen to testimonies, review the evidence, and evaluate the proposed consent decree (see **Fig. 1B$_3$**). One expert consultant observed that the judge had to be "a dispassionate person, so that they're not encumbered by what it's going to cost the State of New Hampshire to fix the system. What they are looking at is inequality, reasonable disparities...the combined impact of this on human beings and so your [judge] is going to make a decision that is based on equality and human principles." However, he added, "They're going to want to see comparative numbers. They're going to want to say, 'Well, is New Hampshire any worse than Vermont? And are we any worse than any other state in terms of our activity and our treatment of our Medicaid population?'"

Once the consent decree and remedies were approved by the judge, orders were sent to implementers (see **Fig. 1C**) who enacted remedies aimed at improving dental care access for beneficiaries (see **Fig. 1D**). The remedies included proposed increases in dental reimbursement rates, an updated registry of Medicaid dentists, and education about EPSDT dental benefits to both beneficiaries and practitioners. A plaintiff attorney noted that the state HHS commissioner became the main implementer. He explained how dentists or "practitioners were implementers [too]. It was the commissioner who decided how to try to reach out to dentists to get them to participate in the [Medicaid] program. So they had a relationship, in remedies [and] implementation."

Beneficiaries could register new grievances with plaintiff attorneys, leading to the start of another cycle (see **Fig. 1A–D**). The *Hawkins* consent decree ended after 6 years, when the judge determined the improvements were sufficient, even though the state had not met the standards outlined in the consent decree and Medicaid policy; that is, to provide all eligible children with dental care. In *Frew*, beneficiaries refiled grievances. As a *Frew* attorney explained, "there were issues over the years in forcing the terms of the consent decree. That went on for years and years and at one point, the state of Texas tried to get out of the consent decree and the case went to the Supreme Court and [it said] 'No, a deal's a deal. You went to a consent decree and now you have to comply with the terms of it.'" The *Frew* case is ongoing.

DISCUSSION

In this study, the goal was to understand the extent to which research evidence is used and generated in the processes underlying dental Medicaid lawsuits. We focused on 2 EPDST case studies, from New Hampshire and Texas, to identify the actors involved in these processes, points at which research evidence was used and generated, and the relationships between actors and research evidence. There were 4 main findings.

First, dentists had key roles in both cases that required scientific expertise or clinical experience based on an understanding of vulnerable populations. Dentists serving as expert witnesses or consultants provided evidence-based testimonies and potential remedies to address access problems for children in Medicaid. To do this, dentists had to know how to identify and interpret the relevant research literature, articulate gaps in scientific knowledge, extrapolate the clinical and policy relevance of studies, and evaluate the strength of scientific evidence for professional guidelines. These advanced science literacy skills are not being adequately addressed in the US predoctoral dental school curricula and should be strengthened through competencies.[25]

Dentists serving as practitioner witnesses testified mainly on the day-to-day difficulties they encountered with the Medicaid program, with most grievances focusing on low reimbursement rates and administrative barriers to dentist participation. Past work highlights the importance of dental Medicaid reimbursement rates in improving dental care use for children, but even in states with the highest reimbursement rates, large proportions of children in Medicaid still fail to see a dentist.[26,27] Thus, reimbursement rates alone are unlikely to boost and sustain utilization unless other barriers to care are addressed. These include attributes of the Medicaid program, such as generosity of benefits (eg, primary molar sealants) and policies that are inconsistent with professional guidelines (eg, recommending first dental visits by age 3 years instead of age 1 year), as well as patient-level factors, such as perceptions that dentists and dental offices are unwelcoming, lack of transportation, and inflexible work schedules.[25,28,29] Cultural sensitivity training for dentists was part of *Frew* consent decree remedies but it is unclear whether this training made a meaningful difference in the way dentists practiced or in beneficiaries' perceptions of dentists. Public health coursework coupled with sensitivity training early in dental school could help students understand that improving access to care requires more than market-based approaches, and reinforce the importance of empathy and flexibility when serving families and children from lower socioeconomic backgrounds.[30]

Second, most research evidence in the 2 cases was newly generated. Existing data sources, such as publications based on analyses of data from national surveys or other state Medicaid programs, were used to frame the problem (eg, barriers to dental care exist for children in Medicaid) and provide a rationale for solutions (eg, sealants reduce disease, preventive dental care is cost-effective). In *Frew*, attorneys used existing data from 416 reports. In *Hawkins*, New Hampshire claims data were procured and analyzed. There are 2 explanations. First, there was a need to establish baseline metrics that did not exist, which were required to track progress. For claims-based measures, utilization trends were assessed over time because this information was not available. However, because of cost and time constraints, there was little or no emphasis on clinical metrics in both cases. By design, this limited the measurable efforts to improve utilization. Use of dental care may play a role in promoting oral health, but by itself dental care is insufficient in preventing disease. Given the paucity of evidence on benefits associated with dental visits, both consent decrees remedies may have missed opportunities to implement additional Medicaid program reforms aimed at reducing disease, boosting health outcomes, and improving the quality of life for children.[31,32] For instance, the consent decrees could have included assurances that resources would be allocated to support implementation of new community-based demonstration projects aimed at dental disease prevention in Medicaid-enrolled children. As an example, a home visitor program could have focused on teaching parents to brush their infants' teeth with fluoridated toothpaste and to only put water into baby bottles at night. Other possibilities include programs to improve use of fluoridated toothpastes and to reduce added sugar intake.[33,34] Prospective data collection would be a central feature of such demonstration projects, to show the effects of such programs, and would form the basis for subsequent evidence-based policymaking. Beneficial demonstration projects could be disseminated statewide to serve all children in Medicaid. Incorporating demonstration projects with formal evaluations as part of consent decree remedies is a promising strategy that could help states improve oral health outcomes for Medicaid enrollees.

There may also have been a geopolitical need to use local data based on the misperception that local problems make external studies nongeneralizable to local conditions. The focus groups and surveys conducted in the 2 states did not result in substantively new information. Most of the findings derived from these efforts were available in the published literature.[4,26,35,36] At the same time, local data may be critical in getting parties to understand the problem, build consensus, and problem solving.

Third, the conceptual model helps to further delineate the role of dentists in Medicaid lawsuits. Dentists were involved in all phases of the lawsuit, from interpreting beneficiaries' grievances on behalf of attorneys, analyzing and interpreting data used to draft the consent decree, testifying during hearings, and implementing remedies as ordered by the judge. This indicates that dentists are not passive bystanders in the legal and health policymaking processes. At times, dentists play critical roles in information brokering between beneficiaries and attorneys, or attorneys and judges.[37] There are specific responsibilities associated with brokering and skills needed in evidence-based policymaking, including knowing how to objectively interpret scientific findings and data, understanding when clinical guidelines and remedies are evidence-based (and when they are not) and the strength of the evidence, and being able to accurately communicate this information to policymakers.[38,39]

An example illustrating the importance of these skills relates to a recent publication on early preventive dental visits for children in Medicaid. This study reported that early visits were not associated with less dental disease and were not cost-savings.[32] These findings are inconsistent with the study that an interviewed attorney cited on the cost-effectiveness of early preventive dental care, which has not been replicated since it was published in 2004.[40] Most practicing dentists believe early visits are important but may not understand that there is weak empirical evidence on the value of prevention. This does not imply that prevention is meaningless. It is an indication that science has not caught up to clinical practice, and underscores the importance of evidence-based dental practice that balances science, craft knowledge, and other factors.[41] High-quality brokering and policymaking requires dentists to understand these nuances and to be able to communicate them to the public. These skills are especially important in the current political climate in which citizens, journalists, and policy-makers are increasingly questioning the value of public expenditures, including health care spending, and alternative facts are used to justify policy decisions.[42]

One way to produce dentists with adequate knowledge-brokering skills is to give pre- and post-doctoral dental students formal opportunities in engage in policy research and advocacy. Students should have the chance to analyze data and publish findings in the peer-reviewed literature. These research experiences should be built on formal coursework in epidemiology, statistics, health policy, research methodology, and other public health topics. Students should find opportunities to present findings to local, state, and federal policymakers and advocate on dental issues to the public in hearings, meetings, and editorial pages. These experiences could culminate in a certificate in dental health policymaking.

Finally, the study underscores the ultimate goals of dental Medicaid lawsuits against states brought forth by marginalized populations; that is, individual and collective social justice, and raises the question of the degree to which justice was actually served. At the individual level, reparations for the named plaintiffs were limited to attorney fees and the promise that families would receive support services so their children could access dental care guaranteed to them under EPSDT. There was no financial or symbolic compensation for the time off from work parents may have taken to search for a Medicaid dentist, the multiple evenings spent waiting in hospital emergency rooms for a physician to provide the child suffering from toothaches with nondefinitive treatment in the form of antibiotics, or for the learning that failed to take place in the classroom because the child in dental pain could not concentrate. Not all of these consequences of untreated tooth decay are directly attributable to inadequate access to dental care but in a health delivery system that blocks the disadvantaged from accessing dental care services that are guaranteed by law, the health care system is at least partially responsible.

In terms of collective social justice, states with a history of dental consent decrees may be able to boost dental utilization rates in the short term, but large proportions of Medicaid-enrolled children still do not utilize care. For instance, in New Hampshire, 24.4% of Medicaid enrollees under age 21 years had an annual dental visit in 2002 during the pre-consent decree period.[43] Based on the most recent published data from 2011, the rate is 60%, which is only slightly higher than the national state-level average for children in Medicaid.[44] Furthermore, some families in Medicaid continue to have problems finding dental care for their children, which motivated the refiling of grievances in Texas. This is a particular concern because it is taking place after initial consent decree remedies have been implemented and at a time when the state Medicaid dental program is being closely scrutinized. How far programs regress in the post-consent decree is unknown and open for empirical evaluation. As stated previously, it is unclear whether consent decrees have meaningfully improved the oral health status of children in these states. These unresolved questions bring into question the parameters in which collective social justice is framed and whether the approach taken in dental Medicaid consent decrees needs to be scrutinized and revamped. At this time, evidence-based approaches offer the greatest opportunity to improve the oral health and make a difference in the lives of children in Medicaid.

Future research should identify the conditions that foster use of research evidence in dental Medicaid lawsuits and whether use of high-quality research evidence improves oral health outcomes of Medicaid-enrolled children. In addition, there is a need to evaluate how researchers in dentistry and public health can better facilitate communication of study findings to attorneys and health scholars. The traditional mode of publishing in peer-reviewed journals and presenting at academic conferences may not be a sufficient method of knowledge transfer. Dental researchers could work with media experts and health journalists to disseminate research findings to a broader audience. Media outlets like the New York Times have special sections, like Gray Matter, for academic researchers to communicate findings to non-researchers.

This study is among the first known studies to examine Medicaid dental lawsuits to understand how research evidence is used and generated in the policymaking process. This study is an important step in understanding the role dental researchers and clinicians have in communicating evidence and formulating health policies that affect publicly insured children. However, there are 3 main limitations. First, we selected 2 states as case studies, which means that our conceptual model may not be generalizable to all states with a dental consent decree history. Second, the study focused on archived materials from the original filing to consent decree approval, limiting the scope of analysis to the first few years of litigation in a process lasting decades. Third, the cases were initially filed in the 1990s, which limited the number of individuals we were able to recruit. In particular, we had hoped to include beneficiaries as part of the key informant interviews but were unable to locate them.

In summary, dental researchers and clinicians play a critical role in dental Medicaid lawsuits aimed at improving the dental care delivery system for vulnerable children. Future efforts should continue to focus on developing strategies to incorporate the highest-quality research evidence into consent decree remedies to ensure that children can also have the opportunity to benefit from dental disease prevention and improvements in quality-of-life and overall health.

REFERENCES

1. Maserejian NN, Trachtenberg F, Link C, et al. Underutilization of dental care when it is freely available: a prospective study of the New England children's amalgam trial. J Public Health Dent 2008;68(3):139–48.

2. Greenberg BJ, Kumar JV, Stevenson H. Dental case management: increasing access to oral health care for families and children with low incomes. J Am Dent Assoc 2008;139(8):1114–21.

3. Capilouto E. The dentist's role in access to dental care by Medicaid recipients. J Dent Educ 1988;52(11):647–52.

4. Lam M, Riedy CA, Milgrom P. Improving access for Medicaid-insured children: focus on front-office personnel. J Am Dent Assoc 1999;130(3):365–73.

5. Kenny GM, Ko G, Ormond BA. Gaps in prevention and treatment: dental care for low-income children. Washington, DC: The Urban Institute, National Survey of America's Families; 2000. Series B, No.B-15.

6. Mofidi M, Rozier RG, King RS. Problems with access to dental care for Medicaid-insured children: what caregivers think. Am J Public Health 2002;92(1):53–8.

7. Davis MM, Hilton TJ, Benson S, et al. Unmet dental needs in rural primary care: a clinic-, community-, and practice-based research network collaborative. J Am Board Fam Med 2010;23(4):514–22.

8. Perkins J. Fact sheet: Medicaid EPSDT case trends and docket. Carrboro: NC: National Health Law Program; 2014. Available at: http://www.healthlaw.org/publications/search-publications/EPSDT-Case-Trends-Docket#.V0xTw5MrLVo/. Accessed December 7, 2016.

9. Macintyre S, Chalmers I, Horton R, et al. Using evidence to inform health policy: case study. BMJ 2001;322(7280):222–5.

10. Contandriopoulos D, Lemire M, Denis JL, et al. Knowledge exchange processes in organizations and policy arenas: a narrative systematic review of the literature. Milbank Q 2010;88(4):444–83.

11. Leslie LK, Maciolek S, Biebel K, et al. Exploring knowledge exchange at the research–policy–practice interface in children's behavioral health services. Adm Policy Ment Health 2014;41(6):822–34.

12. Tseng V. The uses of research in policy and practice. Soc Policy 2012;26(2):1–15.

13. Mitton C, Adair CE, McKenzie E, et al. Knowledge transfer and exchange: review and synthesis of the literature. Milbank Q 2007;85(4):729–68.

14. Davies H, Nutley S, Walter I. Why 'knowledge transfer' is misconceived for applied social research. J Health Serv Res Policy 2008;13(3):188–90.

15. Gehshan S, Snyder A. Why public policy matters in improving access to dental care. Dent Clin North Am 2009;53(3):573–89.

16. Hathaway KL. An introduction to oral health care reform. Dent Clin North Am 2009;53(3):561–72.

17. Bogenschneider K, Corbett T. Evidence-based policymaking: insights from policy-minded researchers and research minded policymakers. New York: Routledge; 2010.

18. Bowen S, Zwi AB. Pathways to "evidence-informed" policy and practice: a framework for action. PLoS Med 2005;2(7):e166.

19. Wang IW, editor. Docket information and court filings. CA: Berkeley: Berkeley Law Library; 2011. Available at: https://www.law.berkeley.edu/library/dynamic/guide.php?id=95. Accessed December 7, 2016.

20. Kerr OS. How to read a legal opinion: a guide for new law students. Green Bag 2007;11(2):51–63.

21. Administrative Office of the United States. Public access to court electronic records (PACER). Washington, DC: Administrative Office of the United States; 2016. Available at: https://www.pacer.gov/. Accessed December 07, 2016.

22. Miles MB, Huberman AM. Qualitative data analysis: an expanded sourcebook. 2nd edition. Thousand Oaks (CA): Sage; 1994.

23. Canadian Health Services Research Foundation (CHSRF). Health services research and evidence-based decision making. Ottawa (Ontario): CHSRF; 2000.

24. Hsieh HF, Shannon SE. Three approaches to qualitative content analysis. Qual Health Res 2005;15(9):1277–88.

25. Nowak AJ, Quiñonez RB. Visionaries or dreamers? The story of infant oral health. Pediatr Dent 2011;33(2):144–52.

26. Decker SL. Medicaid payment levels to dentists and access to dental care among children and adolescents. JAMA 2011;306(2):187–93.

27. Hakim RB, Babish JD, Davis AC. State of dental care among Medicaid-enrolled children in the United States. Pediatrics 2012;130(1):5–14.

28. Chi DL, Singh J. Reimbursement rates and policies for primary molar pit-and-fissure sealants across state Medicaid programs. J Am Dent Assoc 2013; 144(11):1272–8.

29. Straub-Morarend CL, Wankiiri-Hale CR, Blanchette DR, et al. Evidence-based practice knowledge, perceptions, and behavior: a multi-institutional, cross-sectional study of a population of U.S. dental students. J Dent Educ 2016; 80(4):430–8.

30. Wagner JA, Redford-Badwal D. Dental students' beliefs about culture in patient care: self-reported knowledge and importance. J Dent Educ 2008;72(5):571–6.

31. Chi DL, Momany ET, Mancl LA, et al. Dental homes for children with autism: a longitudinal analysis of Iowa Medicaid's I-smile program. Am J Prev Med 2016;50(5): 609–15.

32. Blackburn J, Morrisey MA, Sen B. Outcomes associated with early preventive dental care among Medicaid-Enrolled Children in Alabama. JAMA Pediatr 2017;171(4):335–41.

33. Gray-Burrows KA, Day PF, Marshman Z, et al. Using intervention mapping to develop a home-based parental-supervised toothbrushing intervention for young children. Implement Sci 2016;11:61.

34. Jancey JM, Dos Remedios Monteiro SM, Dhaliwal SS, et al. Dietary outcomes of a community based intervention for mothers of young children: a randomised controlled trial. Int J Behav Nutr Phys Act 2014;11:120.

35. Logan HL, Catalanotto F, Guo Y, et al. Barriers to Medicaid participation among Florida dentists. J Health Care Poor Underserved 2015;26(1):154–67.

36. Al Agili DE, Bronstein JM, Greene-McIntyre M. Access and utilization of dental services by Alabama Medicaid-enrolled children: a parent perspective. Pediatr Dent 2005;27(5):414–21.

37. Langeveld K, Stronks K, Harting J. Use of a knowledge broker to establish healthy public policies in a city district: a developmental evaluation. BMC Public Health 2016;16:271.

38. Bornbaum CC, Kornas K, Peirson L, et al. Exploring the function and effectiveness of knowledge brokers as facilitators of knowledge translation in health-related settings: a systematic review and thematic analysis. Implement Sci 2015;10:162.

39. Neal JW, Neal ZP, Kornbluh M, et al. Brokering the research-practice gap: a typology. Am J Community Psychol 2015;56(3–4):422–35.

40. Savage MF, Lee JY, Kotch JB, et al. Early preventive dental visits: effects on subsequent utilization and costs. Pediatrics 2004;114(4):e418–23.

41. Tonelli MR. Integrating evidence into clinical practice: an alternative to evidence-based approaches. J Eval Clin Pract 2006;12(3):248–56.

42. Merino JG, Jha A, Loder E, et al. Standing up for science in the era of Trump. BMJ 2017;356:j775.

43. Chi D, Milgrom P. Preventive dental service utilization for Medicaid-enrolled children in New Hampshire: a comparison of care provided by pediatric dentists and general dentists. J Health Care Poor Underserved 2009;20(2):458–72.

44. New Hampshire Tool for State Dental Plan. Oral Health Action Plan Template for Medicaid and CHIP Programs. Available at: http://www.medicaid.gov/medicaid/benefits/downloads/sohap-new-hampshire.pdf. Accessed March 1, 2017.

Index

Note: Page numbers of article titles are in **boldface** type.

A

Acculturation, and oral health interventions for children and families, 556–559
  definition of, 549–550
  impact of, on oral health of immigrant children, 551–555
  measurement of, 550
American Academy of Pediatric Dentistry, and people with special health care needs, 573

B

Bacteria transmission, maternal behaviors influencing, 485
  mutans streptococci virulence and, 485
Behavioral factors, affecting maternal oral health and early childhood caries, 485
Biological factors, affecting maternal oral health and early childhood caries, 484

C

CAMBRA tool, caries risk assessment using, 505, 506
Caries, early childhood, 484, 590–591
    and precision health care, 619–620
    bacteria transmission and, 485
    community health workers and, 595
    dental treatments in, 592–593
      medical, 592
      surgical or reparative/retorative, 592–593
    diabetes educators and, 594
    dietitian nutritionists and, 594–595
    family-level behavioral interventions and, 591
    genetic regulation and endophenotypes, 621
    genome-wide association evidence and, 620–621
    health education specialists and, 594
    heritability, and genetic studies, 620
    medical social workers and, 593–594
    nonconventional health workers and, 593–596
    public health professionals and, 595–596
    risk of, prenatal factors affecting, 484–485
  management and control of, during pregnancy, 468–471
  social determinants of, 590
Caries management protocol, for 0-2 year olds, 505, 507–510
Caries risk assessment, using CAMBRA tool, 505, 506
Childhood, early, oral health care in, steps to advance, 622

Childhood (*continued*)
    vision for, 622–623
    precision dentistry in, **619–625**
Children, African refugee, oral health and, 554–555
  Asian, oral health perceptions of, 554
  immigrant, in United States, 550–551
    oral health of, impact of acculturation on, 551–555
  Latino, oral health knowledge and behaviors of, 551–552
    oral health utilization by, 552–553
  of ethnic minorities, delivery of oral health care to, 555–556
  oral health care of, study of, 578–581
  oral health of. See *Oral health, pediatric.*
  oral health team for, expansion of, 580
  traditional dental team for, 578–579
  with special health care needs, consequences of, 566
    definitions of, 565
    functional difficulties among, 572
    future research in, 574
    impact of conditions of, 567–569
    impact on daily activities, 570, 571
    interventions focusing on, **565–576**
    oral health outcomes in, 568–569
    percentage by age, 567
    percentage by race/ethnicity, 569
    percentage by sex, 568
    percentage poverty status, 568
    provision of oral health care for, 571–573
    qualifying criteria, 566–567
    surveys of, 565–566
    unmet dental needs of, 570
children, oral health of, action steps to improve, 598, 599
Community dental health coordinator, 580
Community health workers, for children at risk for caries, 595

D

Dental care, of pregnant women, 504–505
Dental-focused interprofessional interventions, pediatric, **589–606**
    for delivery of better care, 596–600
    to improve oral health of young children, 600–601
Dental hygienists, for care of children, 578–579
Dental intervention, clinical, for children at risk for caries, 597–598
Dental team, traditional, for children, 578–579
Dental therapists, for care of children, 579–580
Dentistry, precision, in early childhood, **619–625**
Dentists, general, for care of children, 578
Dentition, development of, and health behaviors, 534, 536
Diabetes educators, certified, for children at risk for caries, 594
Dietitian nutritionists, registered, for children at risk for caries, 594–595
Disease transmission, intergenerational, method of, 485–486
Diseases, commom, people affected by, worldwide, 534, 535

E

Early and Periodic Screening, Diagnostic, and Treatment program of Medicaid. See *EPSDT*.
EPSDT, Frew and Hawkins lawsuits, actions of, timeline for, 629–630
 case docket documents for, 628, 631
 claims of, 628
 descriptions and roles of actors in, 633
 questions in, 632–639
 relationship between actors and research evidence in, 636–637
 results of, 632–639
 script for key informants' interviews in, 631–632

F

Fluoride, topical, availability of, 607–608
 for prevention of tooth decay, 607, 608
 refusal of, and oral health inequalities, 610
  building scientific evidence to address, 613
  by parent for children, **607–617**
  clinical strategies to manage, 611–613
  defining and conceptualizing of, 608–609
  evidence-based interventions in, 610–611
  measurement gaps, 609
  reasons for, 609–610
Fluoride varnish, 580–581

G

Genetic studies, in heritability of early childhood caries, 620
Genome-wide association evidence, in early childhood caries, 620–621

H

Health care, precision, early childhood caries and, 619–620
Health care needs, special, children with. See *Children, with special health care needs*.
Health education specialists, certified, for children at risk for caries, 594
Healthy People 2020, and factors impacting health, 590–591

I

Intervention studies, in prevention of disease, strategies for, 506–511
 maternal, postdelivery, in disease transmission and caries in children, 487–504
  prenatal, in disease transmission and caries in children, 487, 488–494

L

Lawsuits, Medicaid class action lawsuits dental, screening, diagnostic, and treatment, **627–644**
Lay health workers, in health promotion and disease prevention, 597
 in risk groupdisease management, 597

M

Medicaid, Early and Periodic Screening, Diagnostic, and Treatment program of. See *EPSDT.*
Medicaid class action lawsuits, dental, screening, diagnostic, and treatment, **627–644**
Medical social workers, for children at risk for caries, 593–594
Mutans streptococci virulence, bacteria transmission and, 485

N

Nurse-dietitian team, 580
Nutritionists, dietitian, registered, for children at risk for caries, 594–595

O

Odontogenesis, genomic control of, 621–622
Oral care, of infant, parent/caregiver self-management goals for, 505, 511
Oral care protocol, infant, six-step, 505
Oral health, and health disparities, socio-ecological model of influence on, 534–537, 538
    generational differences in, 540, 541–542
    maternal, prenatal factors affecting, 484–485
    pediatric, access to dental care and workforce issues, 525
        action steps to improve, 598, 599
        conceptional frameworks of, 534–537, 538
        culture/ethnicity/race as influence on, 525
        family function and structure and, 522–523
        future possibilities and research directions in, 543–546
        future research directions to improve, 600–601
        health behaviors and, 523–524
        improvement of, research directions for, 526–527
        influences on, 540, 544–545
        intergenerational and social interventions to improve, **533–548**
        intergenerational influences on, 537–539
        intergenerational interventions in, 540
        social determinants of, **519–532**
        social environment/social capital and, 524
        social interventions and, 540–542
        socioeconomic status and, 520–522
        views of older adults on, 539–540
    prenatal, finance system, 476–477
        interprofessional collaborative training and practice for, 472–476
        intrastructure by state, 472, 473–475
        system intervention for, 471–477
Oral health interventions, during pregnancy, **467–481**
    for individual pregnant woman, 468
    pediatric minority, acculturation and, **549–563**
Oral health outcomes, of child, prenatal maternal factors, intergenerational transmission of disease and, **483–518**
Oral health traits, genomic basis of, 622
Oral hygiene behaviors, pregnant and postpartem women's, studies on, 512

P

Parent/caregiver, refusal of fluoride for children, **607–617**
  self-management goals for infant oral care, 505, 511
Pediatric dental-focused interprofessional interventions, **589–606**
  for delivery of better care, 596–600
  to improve oral health of young children, 600–601
Pediatric workforce issues, 577–588
  future research in, 581–582
Pediatric workforce team, 578–579
"People First" language, in reference to with disabilities, 572
Periodontal health, management of, during pregnancy, 471
Pregnancy, caries management and control during, 468–471
  oral health interventions during, **467–481**
Pregnant women, dental care of, 504–505
Public health personnel, full population intervention by, 597
Public health professionals, certified, for children at risk for caries, 595–596

S

Socioeconomic status, affecting maternal oral health and early childhood caries, 485

T

Tooth decay, socio-ecological model of, 534, 537

Moving?

Make sure your subscription moves with you!

To notify us of your new address, find your **Clinics Account Number** (located on your mailing label above your name), and contact customer service at:

Email: journalscustomerservice-usa@elsevier.com

800-654-2452 (subscribers in the U.S. & Canada)
314-447-8871 (subscribers outside of the U.S. & Canada)

Fax number: 314-447-8029

Elsevier Health Sciences Division
Subscription Customer Service
3251 Riverport Lane
Maryland Heights, MO 63043

*To ensure uninterrupted delivery of your subscription, please notify us at least 4 weeks in advance of move.

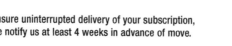
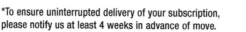

Printed and bound by CPI Group (UK) Ltd, Croydon, CR0 4YY

03/10/2024

01040395-0018